Physiology for sportspeople

For my girls and my parents

Physiology for sportspeople

A *serious user's guide to the body*

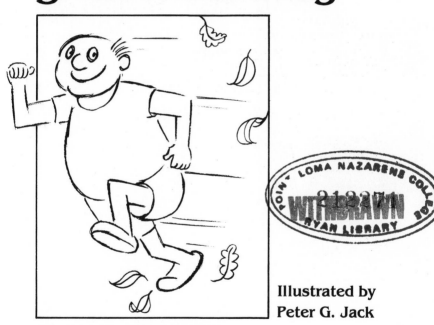

Illustrated by
Peter G. Jack

Peter G. Bursztyn

Manchester University Press
Manchester and New York
Distributed exclusively in the USA and Canada by St. Martin's Press

Copyright © Peter Bursztyn 1990

Published by Manchester University Press
Oxford Road, Manchester M13 9PL, UK
and Room 400, 175 Fifth Avenue,
New York, NY 10010, USA

*Distributed exclusively in the USA and Canada
by* St. Martin's Press, Inc.,
175 Fifth Avenue, New York, NY 10010, USA

British Library cataloguing in publication data
Bursztyn, Peter
  Physiology for sportspeople.
  1. Sports & games. Physiological aspects
  I. Title
  612.044

Library of Congress cataloging in publication data
Bursztyn, Peter.
   Physiology for sportspeople: a serious user's guide to the body/
Peter G. Bursztyn: illustrated by Peter G. Jack.
      p.   cm.
   Includes bibliographical references (p.   ) and index.
   ISBN 0-7190-3086-2 (hardback). — ISBN 0-7190-3087-0 (pbk.)
   1. Sports—Physiological aspects.   I. Title.
RC1235.887   1990
612'.044—dc.20   90-6308

Typeset in Hong Kong
by Best-set Typesetter Ltd.

Printed in Great Britain
by Bell & Bain Limited, Glasgow

Contents:

Contents

Acknowledgements

I was taught physiology at McGill University in Montreal by a group of academics dedicated to their discipline, who managed to instil some of that dedication and love of the subject into me. Since I moved away from Canada very soon after graduation, my memories of Professor F.C. MacIntosh, and those of his staff who taught me are memories of the youthful, lively people they were nearly thirty years ago. I prefer to remember them that way. I am indebted to my supervisor, R.I. Birks, who insisted on honesty in research and meticulous preparation for lectures. When I first elected to read Physiology, Kay Terroux doubted that I had the level of commitment she felt I required, and admitted me into the department reluctantly. I hope that she would not regret her decision, were she still alive. Duncan Cameron, who both helped and terrified students for decades also lives only in memory now.

Although I was taught a great deal of physiology during my eight years at McGill, I realised how much I still had to learn when I faced my first class of medical students in Nairobi. In a sense, those Kenyan students (the first medical class in Kenya) taught me more than I had ever learned before. Their questions and those of their successors made a proper physiologist of me. On the way, they forced me to express myself in straightforward sentences which students can understand. Meanwhile David Horrobin, the head of department, spent four years trying to turn me into a keen observer and a philosopher.

I spent fourteen years at the University of Southampton where I began teaching exercise and environmental physiology. I used these subjects as a vehicle to give students a much needed review while covering new ground. I first thought of writing a book on exercise physiology because a colleague read, and praised, some of the notes I gave out to the students. Alan Thomas does not know that he planted the idea for this book, but I am grateful. The fledgling book was further encouraged by Barbara York who asked me so many questions that I handed her an early version of the metabolism chapter to help her out. She was kind enough to offer me praise when I badly needed it.

I received valuable assistance in the area of biochemistry from Ian Giles and I thank him for the time he spent with me. I would also like to thank Steve Wooton for helping me understand muscle metabolism.

I was fortunate to meet Peter Jack. I originally hoped that he would do anatomical drawings. However, he proved to be an adept cartoonist and was soon decorating graphs and tables as well. If this book is a success, a large portion of the credit will be his.

I am particularly grateful to John Harrison for the many insights he offered me on exercise testing. He was kind enough to read a number of chapters and to offer a great deal of constructive criticism. Niall Horn and I had many physiological arguments over the years to our mutual benefit. He too has read much of this book and made many useful suggestions. It was only after I left Southampton that I realised how very generous and helpful these ex-colleagues had been. John has managed to continue helping me from 5000 miles away, via his fax machine!

I must give grudging thanks to the Tory government whose attempts to judge academic endeavour using financial measures made life sufficiently uncomfortable that I was forced to write this book in self defence. Eventually, any success this book enjoys will have come too late. My recent resignation from the University of Southampton was in protest against the use of research grant income as a yardstick to gauge academic achievement.

Finally, I must mention the role this book has played in making me fat and unfit. Now that it is finished, I have been pedalling to work — a round trip of twenty miles — several times each week. This has, unfortunately, proven to me that vigorous exercise by itself cannot cause weight loss (Chapter 10). At any rate, I am now fit and fat.

P.G.B.
September 1989, Barrie, Ontario

CHAPTER ONE

Introduction to exercise physiology

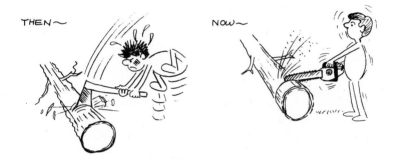

introduction

In the richer countries of the world physical work as a part of employment is disappearing. Over a century ago, the industrial revolution mechanised many of the repetitive tasks in various industries (textile weaving, mining, steel fabrication, etc.) which had required human muscle to perform. The mechanisation of transport gradually brought effortless transport and personal travel within the reach of most people. In the first sixty years of this century, powered tools have taken much of the effort out of all manner of work including farming, road paving, building, baking, carpentry, and most assembly tasks. More recently, domestic mechanisation has replaced muscular effort in the kitchen, the garden and the laundry, and very few people now need to move either coal or ashes to heat their homes. Many people even pay professional sportsmen to play games on their behalf!

The mechanisation of transport has probably had the greatest impact on routine physical activity. Before the Second World War, factory workers had much of their physical labour lightened by machinery, but they still needed to walk or bicycle to work, often quite a long distance. Today, both public transport and car owner-

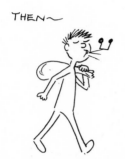

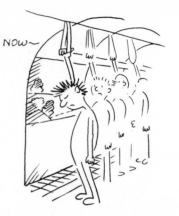

ship are widespread and very few people now expend physical effort in travelling to work.

Emancipation from physical work combined with shorter working hours have made leisure a large and growing industry. For most people, leisure suggests relaxation and relative inactivity. However, a steadily increasing minority devote at least part of their leisure time to exercise. Some people enjoy the camaraderie and competition of sports and games. Others simply wish to maintain some degree of physical fitness. The fitness and exercise boom is strongly encouraged by manufacturers of sports and fitness equipment, who have tried to erase the sweaty image of exercise, making it more glamourous, attractive, and expensive than ever before. At the same time government agencies, and the medical profession have been saying that physical fitness is "healthy". A growing number of employers believe that they can see productivity and savings in promoting the health of their employees, and have also been advertising the benefits of fitness.

Part of this book is concerned with the supposed benefits of exercise, with respect to psychological well-being, cardiovascular disease, obesity, hypertension, and most recently, osteoporosis. Some of the problems associated with exercise including muscle damage, heart attacks, heat prostration, etc. are described and explained.

However, it is important to keep two facts in mind. Although awareness of exercise and its claimed benefits has grown greatly in the last two decades, only a small minority of the populations of

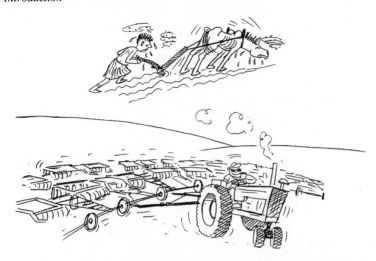

prosperous western countries are physically active, let alone physically fit. Nevertheless, in the 20th century the populations of the western world have experienced an increase in longevity of some 15–20 years. This has happened while there has been a substantial reduction in the amount of actual work that most people have to do.

I do not believe that physical activity and fitness either ward off illness or prolong life. However, I do believe that a reasonable degree of fitness is an important adjunct to the full enjoyment of life.

exercise, co-operation between various organs
To do work, the body requires energy — obtained as food and stored as fat, carbohydrate, and protein. These foods must be oxidised or "burned" to liberate their energy. Hence oxygen must be obtained and delivered, and wastes collected and discarded. Muscular activity must be co-ordinated to produce purposeful motion. The heat produced by oxidising the food must be dissipated. Finally, when activity stops, the body must be returned to its original state, with its energy stores full, ready to go once again.

Obviously, work is the result of muscular shortening acting on the skeleton which converts these contractions into useful movement. However, various systems must co-operate for the body to

3

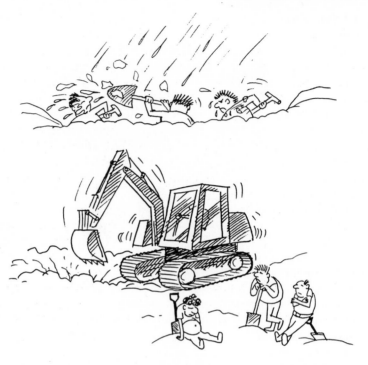

produce work. These include liver and fat tissue to store food energy; metabolism to convert food energy into energy for contraction; lungs to obtain oxygen for metabolism; heart and blood vessels to deliver energy and oxygen to working tissues, to remove waste products and heat; and a thermoregulatory system to maintain a normal body temperature by getting rid of the heat. In addition, the brain must co-ordinate movement, water resources are mustered, repairs and maintenance are carried out, wastes excreted ...

Exercise physiology is concerned with the performance, limitations, co-ordination, training, and development of these systems. This book considers only those systems most directly concerned with exercise.

exercise, physiological limitations and improvement
The more physically fit a person is, the more acutely aware they are of their limitations. Which physiological systems tend to limit performance and why? What are the differences between sprinters

4

and endurance athletes? Do the same systems limit performance in both cases?

Part of this book will concern itself with the physiological changes which accompany training. No attempt is made to suggest training programmes. However, it is hoped that athletes, aspiring athletes, their teachers and their coaches will begin to understand some of the physiological processes underlying exercise. This should help them to devise and to improve training programmes.

One of the improvement techniques to which athletes have been turning are drugs. These range from everyday stimulants like caffeine (coffee and tea), and relatively benign over-the-counter analgesics or anti-inflammatory preparations. However, they also include banned and dangerous substances such as sex steroids and amphetamines, and very addictive drugs like cocaine. The taking of drugs specifically to improve performance is counter to the spirit of sport. Victory on the athletic field should belong to the sportsman, and not to his/her pharmacist. Moreover, many of the drugs and hormones (synthetic and natural) used to improve performance can damage health, and some have even been blamed for the deaths of athletes who had used them. This subject is thoroughly reviewed and explained, spelling out the effects of various preparations on performance (if any), the mechanism of action (if known), and the dangers associated with them.

It is hoped that this book will help non-athletes come to terms with their performance. Alchemy was discredited by modern chemistry. Similarly, modern physiology can be used to explain why training is not able to transform everybody, however determined, into championship material. Some individuals are genetically suited to long distance running and are unlikely to ever become competitive in the hammer throw, while most of us will never attain stardom in any physical activity, whatever effort we put into it. Many years ago the Swedish exercise physiologist, Per Olof Astrand, said "I am convinced that anyone interested in winning Olympic Gold Medals must select his parents very carefully."

the body is a remarkable machine
Many aspects of the body and its performance are humbling. The heart beats 40,000,000 times each year, and in a typical day, pumps fifteen tons of blood. The respiratory system, within a chest whose volume is two gallons, packs a surface area the size of half a tennis court. When working continuously at full power, the

body produces over 1000 watts of heat, and manages to get rid of it, tolerating only a small rise in temperature.

Among the more remarkable properties of the body are that:

1. it is powered by cheap, commonplace fuels,
2. at an efficiency comparable to the very best machines man has ever devised,
3. working with a reliability that Rolls Royce, Boeing, and IBM only dream of attaining, and,
4. on the rare occasions when failure does occur, it possesses a remarkable capacity to repair itself.

As if these features were not enough, the body is also tough, hard to damage and particularly undemanding with respect to maintenance.

The ability of the body to produce a useful work output should not be underestimated. As we all know, the harder one works the shorter is one's endurance. It is difficult to measure the power output of a person engaged in most normal activities such as walking, swimming, sawing, chopping, digging, etc. Instead, measurements are usually made while operating a bicycle-like machine called an ergometer or "work measurer". Thus harnessed, an average man can produce around a quarter of a horsepower or 200 watts for many minutes; while some can carry on at this rate for hours. Over short periods of less than 30 seconds power outputs of one kilowatt are developed. During extremely brief "explosive" activity, such as throwing an object, or swinging an axe, far higher rates of work are possible.

All of these are the province of the exercise physiologist, and it is hoped that this book will be able to introduce and explain this fascinating subject to the lay reader. However, the intention was to produce a book which is both accurate and comprehensive. It is hoped that very few questions to which there are answers have been left unanswered, and that this has been accomplished with a minimum of jargon and abbreviation. Where scientific terms have been used, these are fully explained in the text. For people who miss the explanations by reading this book out of sequence, an extensive glossary is provided. For those who have found the topic fascinating and wish to know more, a reading list is provided.

I hope that you enjoy the subject as much as I have.

CHAPTER TWO

Muscle

Every movement the body carries out is powered by muscle. The body has three types of muscle: skeletal (or striated), cardiac, and smooth. Skeletal muscle is, with a very few exceptions, connected to bones so that muscle shortening or contraction moves the skeleton. Skeletal muscle is the most abundant tissue in the body, making up roughly half the body weight of most people and animals. Most of the meat that we eat is skeletal muscle.

The skeletal muscles operate on bony levers whose fulcrums are the joints. For example, the biceps muscle of the upper arm is attached to the forearm at a point approximately 1/10 of the distance between the elbow joint and the hand (Fig. 2.1). If a weight of 10 kg is held in the hand, the force which the muscle must exert is equivalent to a 100 kg weight hanging from the tendon. All of the human body's levers and fulcrums are arranged to favour speed of movement. This requires the muscles to produce and tendons to transmit very large forces. For example, the achilles tendon of the heel readily copes with loads over one ton.

Smooth muscle, on the other hand, is arranged in tubes or sacs whose contraction squeezes the contents and causes them to flow, or divides the tube into separate compartments so that any flow stops. Smooth muscle is the main constituent of the stomach, intestine, urinary tract, and of the arteries and veins. Both smooth and skeletal muscle can be further classified by their function and characteristics. Cardiac muscle, the third type, makes up the bulk of the heart, and has properties which place it part way between the other two.

Skeletal muscle is of particular interest to the athlete and, being a highly organised tissue, is also simpler to describe than either cardiac or smooth muscle. Skeletal muscle cells are long (10–15 cm) and thin (50–100 μm). They are encased in a semi-permeable membrane which, aside from being a simple wrapping, maintains the internal concentration of solutes (dissolved substances), trans-

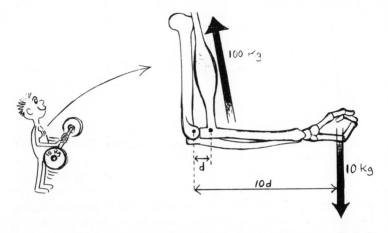

Fig. 2.1 The skeleton is a collection of levers and fulcrums on which the muscles operate to cause movement. The tension developed by a muscle may be many times the weight it supports at the end of a limb.

ports material into and out of the cell, and has a number of other functions as well.

The muscle cell membrane

Living tissue is mostly water, in which salts called electrolytes (because they conduct electricity) are dissolved. In watery solution, electrolytes separate into ions, which are particles carrying either positive or negative charges. Ions move under the influence of an electrical field, thus conducting an electrical current. The composition of the fluids inside and outside the cells differ because ionic pumps within the membrane actively transport certain electrolytes. These differences in composition are maintained by the semi-permeable membrane which restricts the movement of some of the dissolved ions.

the membrane potential

The existence of a semi-permeable membrane separating two fluids with different compositions causes a voltage to appear across the membrane. This voltage, or membrane potential, is a characteristic of all living cells. The resting cell membrane is permeable to (allows the passage of) potassium ions, but not to sodium ions (both positively charged). Moreover, special ion pumps remove sodium from the cell so

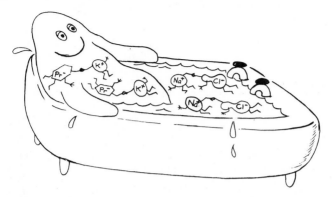

Fig. 2.2 The body's cells contain a solution, the intracellular fluid, rich in potassium (K). They are bathed in the extracellular fluid, a solution rich in sodium (Na) and chloride (Cl) ions. Proteins (Pr) carry most of the negative charges inside cells.

that it is abundant in the fluid outside and scarce inside, while the reverse is true for potassium. Positive and negative charges pair up so that all parts of an electrolyte solution are at the same voltage, and the total number of positive and negative charges in the solution are always equal. Most of the negative charges outside the cell are held on chloride ions, paired with sodium, while most of the negative charges inside cells are held on proteins which are fixed within the cell, and paired with potassium.

Potassium ions try to escape from the cell since they are "crowded" inside while their external concentration is low. As they try to do this, they leave behind "lonely" negative ions (mainly proteins) which are too large to follow, and in muscle are anyhow fixed within the cell. The negative charge created by potassium's attempt to emigrate attracts the ions back, preventing them from moving far (Fig. 2.3). This negative charge inside the cell is the "resting membrane potential", and averages −80 millivolts. The resting membrane potential is mainly determined by the difference in potassium ion concentration across the cell membrane. Since the membrane blocks the passage of sodium ions, these have little effect on the resting membrane potential.

The muscle membrane has one further property. It is electrically insulating and ensures that individual skeletal muscle cells always work independently. By contrast, in heart muscle, patches of the membrane are electrically conducting, ensuring that active muscle cells always stimulate their neighbours. In healthy heart muscle, when one part of the muscle is activated, the whole muscle responds synchronously.

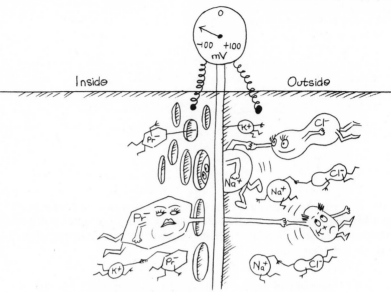

Fig. 2.3 The cell membrane behaves as if it is porous. In the resting membrane, these pores do not normally allow sodium ions through, but potassium ions pass freely.

the action potential

Disturbance of the muscle resting membrane potential by way of a nerve signal is the normal means of stimulating and activating a cell. The nerve signal excites the muscle cell membrane by releasing a chemical (called a neurotransmitter) from the nerve ending. This chemical, acetylcholine, travels across the tiny gap between the nerve and the muscle (the synapse) where it causes a short circuit, dropping the voltage and depolarising the membrane locally. This triggers a widespread depolarisation, the action potential, which travels the length of the muscle cell in both directions.

During the action potential, the characteristics of the membrane change dramatically. It suddenly becomes far more permeable to sodium ions than to potassium. (Fig. 2.3 suggests that the membrane has holes or pores which prevent larger ions from crossing. This is not true and membrane permeability is more complex than this.) Now the sodium ions, "crowded" outside the cell and scarce inside, attempt to enter. Since they move far more rapidly than their partners, the chloride ions, they leave "lonely" negative charges behind, making the inside of the cell positive by about 40 millivolts for the brief instant of the action potential.

The action potential lasts only 1–2 milliseconds in nerve cells, about 10 milliseconds in the cells of skeletal muscle, and over 100 milliseconds in heart muscle. Immediately after the action potential, the membrane reverts to blocking the passage of sodium, and its voltage returns to the normal resting value of −80 millivolts.*

Inside the muscle cell — the contraction machinery

Let us dissect the whole muscle to magnify and look at the contraction machinery. Individual muscles are wrapped up in a tough sheath of connective tissue. This is slippery, allowing adjacent muscles to glide against each other with little friction. The muscle itself is made up of bundles (fasciculi) of single muscle fibres or cells (Fig. 2.4). These bundles are also wrapped in connective tissue. Finally, the individual muscle cells are surrounded by very thin connective tissue in addition to their cell membrane.

Within the membrane, the skeletal muscle cell is packed with strands of two kinds of protein, actin and myosin. Myosin is like a golf club. The shafts of several hundred strands of myosin are bundled together forming a thick filament, with their heads spiralling around the bundle (Fig. 2.5). The myosin filament is double ended, smooth in the middle, with the myosin heads arranged around either end. Meanwhile, strands of actin pair up to form thin filaments in a hexagonal array, with six actin filaments surrounding each end of the thick myosin filament (Fig. 2.4). The actin filaments penetrate a sheet of material called a Z-plate, and surround another myosin filament on its other side.

Groups of thin actin filaments surround both ends of every thick myosin filament. Bundles of such units (sarcomeres) are the smallest functional subdivisions of the contractile mechanism. Although the individual filaments are too thin to be seen using an ordinary microscope (but are seen with an electron microscope), their presence gives the sarcomere a distinctly banded appearance (Fig. 2.4). Sarcomeres are attached end to end by their Z-plates in a long chain forming a myofibril. The alternating bands make the

---

* (The electric eel, among other electric fish, has a specialised electric organ which sums the voltages of many membranes together, like cells in a car battery. When the fish activates this organ with acetylcholine, the action potentials add together, giving rise to over 500 volts which can kill or stun either prey or predator.)

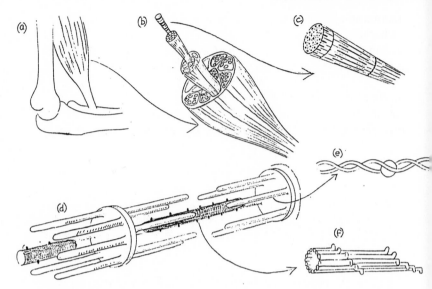

Fig. 2.4 (a) muscle, (b) bundles of muscle fibres (cells), (c) a fibril, which is a bundle of contracting units called (d) the sarcomere, (e) the thin actin filaments which form temporary chemical bonds with (f) the thick myosin filaments.

myofibril look striped and give skeletal muscle its alternative name, striated muscle. Many myofibrils are packed together within the cell membrane to form a muscle fibre, and many fibres, tied together with connective tissue and tendons, make up a muscle.

One other anatomical feature of skeletal muscle is important. There is a set of membranes, the sarcoplasmic reticulum, located within each muscle cell. The function of these membranes is to store calcium ions. When the cell is stimulated, this calcium is released briefly, initiating contraction (Fig. 2.7).

The structure of heart muscle is similar to that of skeletal muscle, except that individual muscle cells are electrically connected to each other, and when one is stimulated, the excitation spreads through the whole organ. Smooth muscle is quite different. It consists of the same proteins as striated muscle, but completely lacks the calcium storage membranes and the regular structure. Neither striations nor sarcomeres can be seen. The filaments are scattered about each cell in a disorganised fashion. This lack of organisation limits strength but gives smooth muscle the ability to work over an astonishingly wide range of muscle length. By comparison, heart muscle is limited to operating over less than 30% of its resting length, and skeletal muscle to about 10%.

the contraction machinery at work

During muscular contraction, the thin filaments slide over the thick filaments, and the sarcomeres shorten, making the muscle

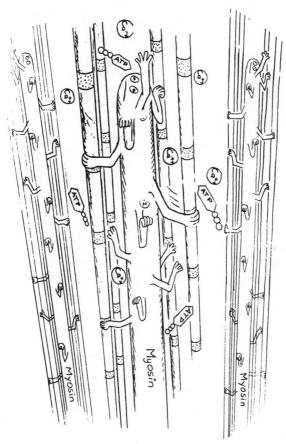

Fig. 2.5 Thick myosin filaments pull themselves along the thin actin filaments to cause muscle shortening or contraction. This process is activated by calcium or Ca^{++} ions (p. 15) released during the action potential, and powered by ATP (Ch. 3).

contract. When calcium ions are released inside the cell (see below), the myosin heads form chemical bonds (cross-bridges) with adjacent positions on the actin filaments. Using energy from ATP (see Ch. 3), the myosin head bends, pulling the actin filament past the myosin filament. Attachment of a fresh ATP breaks the cross-bridge chemical bond. If calcium is still present, new bonds are formed immediately at the next available position. Repetition of this process ratchets the filaments past each other causing the sarcomere to shorten and the muscle to contract.

Forming and breaking a single cross-bridge shortens a sarcomere by just 8 millionths of a millimetre, or by about 0.4%. In theory, during a maximal contraction, this ratcheting process can be repeated by up to fifty times to give a shortening of 20%. Some of this shortening is taken up in tensioning elastic elements within the muscle. In reality the shortening of striated muscle is usually limited to around 10% of the muscle's resting length. This limitation is imposed by the skeleton, which does not allow a muscle to be stretched excessively or to shorten too much — either would reduce the tension developed.

rigor mortis
After death, the absence of oxygen causes the muscle fibres to depolarise, release free calcium, and contract. These contractions are usually not visible because of their disorganised and asynchronous nature. However, when the ATP stores are depleted, the energy to break crossbridges which have formed is no longer available. The actin and myosin remain chemically bonded, giving rise to *rigor mortis*, where the limbs become quite rigid. If a person dies in vigorous exercise (for example, a villain shot while running away) *rigor mortis* develops rapidly because the muscle is already partly depleted of ATP. Eventually, relaxation occurs because the contractile proteins begin to break down through self-digestion. This is the reason why butchers "hang" meat for several days to tenderise it. The presence or absence of *rigor mortis* is one of the clues used by pathologists to ascertain the time of death.

muscle activation or stimulation of the contraction
The contraction process of making and breaking cross-bridges between the myosin and actin filaments is triggered by the presence of calcium within the cell. Normally, there is very little free

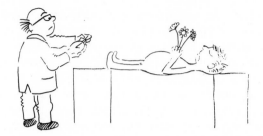

Fig. 2.6 *In rigor mortis the temporary chemical bonds between actin and myosin become permanent because of the absence of ATP. Because of this, the muscle cannot be moved and the body becomes rigid. The state of rigor mortis in the body provides clues to the timing of death.*

calcium inside the cell. Calcium is stored attached to the cell membrane and to a network of intracellular membranes called the sarcoplasmic reticulum. During the action potential, the voltage change causes these membranes to release their stored calcium making it available to trigger the contraction machinery.

When the resting potential is restored, the free calcium is quickly scavenged out of the cell, reattaching itself to the storage sites, ready for the next contraction. The drop in the free calcium concentration in the cell causes relaxation.

One of the differences between smooth muscle and striated muscle is that the former has little or no calcium stored within the cell. Stimulation of the smooth muscle cell initially has no effect. Trains of action potentials allow calcium to enter the smooth

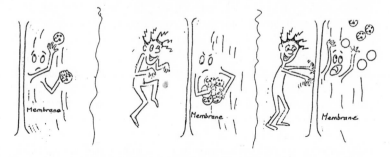

Fig. 2.7 *The resting membrane collects and holds most of the calcium within the cell. The action potential causes the membrane to release calcium which then goes on to activate the contractile mechanism.*

muscle cell from the outside while the membrane is depolarised. The contraction develops gradually as the calcium concentration inside the cell rises. Fortunately, smooth muscle is never in a hurry. In skeletal muscle, calcium is available almost instantly because it is stored close to where it is needed. Cardiac muscle stores some calcium, but the development of tension depends largely on how much calcium enters the cell during its lengthy action potential. Control of calcium entry by adrenalin is the main way in which the strength of cardiac muscle contraction is regulated.

Control of contraction strength

In an individual muscle fibre or cell a contraction is an "all-or-nothing" event — that is, once stimulated, an individual muscle fibre is committed to a contraction. However, in real life we have excellent control of our muscles.

Single muscle fibres are not activated individually. To do so would require a nerve fibre for every muscle fibre, and very thick nerve trunks. Instead, muscle fibres are grouped into motor units containing between 5 and 1000 fibres, each stimulated by a single nerve fibre. The muscle fibres making up each motor unit are not grouped together, but are scattered about the body of the muscle. One method of controlling the tension developed by a muscle is by stimulating varying numbers of motor units. Muscles whose duties are mainly postural (back, leg) have relatively small numbers of large motor units (as few as 100) each with many muscle fibres. These cannot be very finely controlled. The muscles which carry out delicate movements (fingers, eyes, tongue) have a very large number of small motor units (up to 2000 in the eye muscles), and are capable of delicate adjustments in tension.

Another means of controlling the force of contraction is by varying the frequency with which a nerve stimulates its motor unit. A single nerve stimulus results in a brief, weak contraction called a twitch. If a second stimulus follows quickly, a second twitch will occur before the muscle relaxes, and its tension will build on that of its predecessor (Fig. 2.8). Muscles are normally stimulated by bursts of nerve activity lasting several seconds. The resulting contraction is called a tetanus. The faster the frequency of impulses within such a burst, the greater the tension which is developed.

16

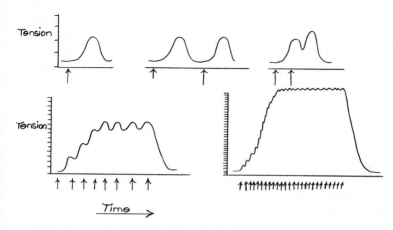

Fig. 2.8 Tension is developed when a muscle is stimulated. A single action potential gives rise to a twitch. The tension produced in twitches can add together. The frequency at which the muscle is stimulated is one way to control the tension it develops. Arrows indicate stimulation.

Slow and fast muscle

Several different types of fibres are found in muscle. The two extreme types are labelled "slow" and "fast", although intermediate types also exist. Fast fibres develop more tension and contract faster than slow fibres. On the other hand, slow fibres have far greater endurance. The intermediate types partly share the features of both. Some of the characteristics of slow and fast fibres are tabulated below:

Table 2.1 *Muscle fibre type*

Property	Fast twitch (white)	Slow twitch (red)
Myoglobin	little	much
Capillary supply	sparse	dense
Fibre diameter	large	small
ATP-splitting enzyme	much	little
Contraction strength	high	low
Metabolism favoured	anaerobic	aerobic
Glycogen content	high	low
Metabolic efficiency	low	high
Fatigue resistance	low	high
Activation threshold	high (hard to activate)	low (easily activated)

"Fast" fibres are twice as fast as "slow" fibres but this is of little importance for most activities. The greater tension of fast fibres comes from their larger diameter, but they are no stronger when corrected for size. The main differences between fibre types relate not to their contraction speed, but to their metabolic properties, and to their blood supply.

slow twitch muscle favours aerobic metabolism

The colour of a muscle comes from both its myoglobin content and the amount of blood in it. Myoglobin is related to haemoglobin, the oxygen transporting pigment in blood. The presence of myoglobin increases the speed with which oxygen diffuses through the muscle tissue. So oxygen diffusion between the capillary and the muscle fibre is faster in red than in white muscle (see p. 94).

Red muscle contains more blood than white because it has a dense network of capillaries. The high capillary density reduces the average diffusion distance between the capillary and the muscle fibre, again improving oxygen transfer in red muscle as compared to white muscle.

Finally, because slow fibres are small, they tend to be closer to their blood supply than are the larger diameter fast fibres. These three properties allow slow fibres to obtain oxygen more rapidly than fast fibres, favouring aerobic metabolism.

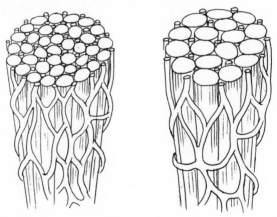

Fig. 2.9 Slow fibres are small, which brings them closer to their blood supply. The large fast fibres tend to have a less generous network of capillaries.

Accordingly, slow fibres contain many mitochondria, the intracellular structures where aerobic metabolism takes place (Ch. 3). Although slow fibres have small stores of glycogen, their generous blood supply allows them to obtain their glucose and fat from the circulation, a very extensive energy resource. Reliance on aerobic metabolism, together with the ability to take up oxygen and nutrients at a high rate from the blood, give the slow fibres their great endurance. The endurance of the body's postural muscles is well known, and the muscles of the back are able to maintain a steady tension for many hours.

fast twitch muscle favours anaerobic metabolism

On the other hand, fast twitch muscle fibres are capable of very high rates of ATP production by glycolysis (anaerobic metabolism). This can supply the high rate of work output often demanded of this type of muscle. The existence locally of large amounts of glycogen give fast muscle fibres the rapid access to energy supplies which they require.

Fast twitch muscle contains few mitochondria, where aerobic metabolism takes place. Consequently, this type of muscle is not capable of high rates of aerobic activity. Only aerobic metabolism uses the lactic acid produced by glycolysis (see Ch. 3), and active fast twitch muscle rapidly "poisons" itself with lactic acid. It also tends to run out of energy quickly by using only 5% of that available in its glycogen (the remainder is not wasted, but is often lost from the slow muscle fibre into the blood, where it may be used by other tissues — Ch. 3). Consequently, the endurance of fast muscle is poor. Its rapid fatiguability is readily demonstrated if you attempt to hold a chair at arm's length for two minutes ...

how are the various muscle types used?

In our bodies, the muscles whose major concern is the maintenance of posture contain a large proportion of slow fibres, and these are organised in large motor units. On the other hand, muscles used mostly for quick, accurate movement are composed mainly of fast fibres, grouped in small motor units.

Of interest to the athlete is the fact that fast fibres are used for maximum or explosive power which will be sustained only for seconds, or minutes at most. These fibres can produce great tension and carry out work at a high rate thanks to their ability to extract energy anaerobically. The muscles of the arm and hand are predominantly composed of fast fibres, although slow fibres are also present.

Slow muscle fibres are used for endurance work, that is, for relatively light work loads which are to be sustained for many minutes or even hours. In particular, the postural muscles of the back are predominantly composed of slow fibres, and some are 90% slow fibres.

A chicken is only capable of brief flight. This is because its flight (breast) muscles are exclusively pale, rapidly fatiguing fast fibres. On the other hand, the duck's breast or flight muscles are dark in colour, reflecting its great endurance in flight. The leg muscles of a chicken are also dark, since this bird is a runner by trade.

can we choose or control which muscle fibres we use?
The degree of effort required largely determines the type of muscle fibre which participates in generating movement. Motor units made up of slow fibres are activated by small neurons (nerve cells), while the large neurons control fast fibre motor units. Since small nerve cells are easier to stimulate than large ones, this means that slow muscle fibres tend to be activated for movement requiring less effort. As more energetic movements are attempted, larger nerve cells tend to be recruited, eventually including those controlling the fast fibres. Of course, the actual proportion of fibre types (recall that there is a spectrum of intermediate types between the fast and slow types) activated also depends on the composition of the whole muscle. Thus, work carried out using the arms would use more fast fibres than leg work because of the relative proportion of fibre types in these limbs.

Fatigue is a complex and incompletely understood process part of which is also dealt with in Ch. 3. The sensation of fatigue can be partly explained by the ease with which the various fibre types are activated. During endurance exercise, the work load is light and the force of contraction is low, so that mainly slow fibres are activated. These endurance fibres are resistant to fatigue. However, when they do tire, limb movement will falter unless fresh, unfatigued fibres are recruited. These "rested" fibres have been quiescent because they are controlled by larger, less easily stimulated nerve cells. To activate these larger nerve cells requires a greater number of nerve signals and thus more mental effort. The increasing mental effort gives a sensation of fatigue. Eventually, when so many muscle fibres are fatigued that accurate movement is no longer possible, not only does the sensation of fatigue become acute, but the chance of injury due to poor co-ordination is greatly increased.

Muscle type and athletic performance

Samples of muscle can be obtained using large biopsy needles which cut out cylinders of tissue (under anaesthetic) for analysis. Using the appropriate microscopic techniques, it is possible to determine the proportion of slow, fast, or intermediate fibres making up that muscle. In the legs of well trained distance runners, 80% of the muscle may be composed of slow fibres. By contrast, sprinters' muscles may be 75% fast fibres. Middle distance runners and jumpers, and sedentary people have leg muscles in which fast and slow fibres are more or less equally represented.

Although the above looks clear, it is only a guide, because there are wide variations within each group. Thus, the muscles of some excellent sprinters and some elite distance runners have approximately equal numbers of slow and fast fibres. The correlation between the fibre population of the leg muscles and the running performance of an athlete is poor. Also, many muscle fibres are intermediate types with the characteristics of both fast and slow fibres and hard to classify. In general, it would be unwise to select a national athletic squad on the basis of biopsy results.

nature or nurture — is heredity or training responsible?
Nevertheless, there is a tendency for sprinters to have fast muscle fibres in their legs. Clearly, children do not obtain muscle biopsies to determine whether they are best suited for sprint or for distance running. Rather, after a period of time it becomes clear that an individual is more successful at one event than another. Since winning is more fun than losing, they tend to specialise in those events in which they are most successful. So, do sprinters have fast fibres in their legs because (a) they were born that way, or (b) because they spent their youth training as sprinters?

The answer is neither exclusively (a) nor (b). In experiments

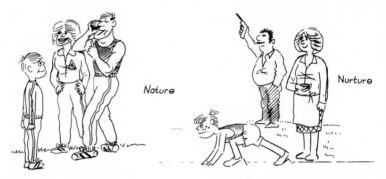

Fig. 2.10 *Children who are sons or daughters of athletes may have received a genetic advantage for certain types of activity from their parents. It is not certain whether training in childhood may alter the proportion of fast and slow muscle fibres, which is not really possible in adulthood.*

where the (fast) muscles of sprinters were biopsied before and after several weeks of endurance training it was found that the numbers of mitochondria in the muscle fibres and their enzyme activity increased, as did the density of capillaries within the muscle. In other words, their fast muscle fibres appeared to become more adept at aerobic work. However, the proportion of muscle fibres which could be classified as either fast or slow remained basically unchanged.

In another study where distance runners were given several weeks of sprint training, their fast muscle fibres showed a greater increase in diameter than did their slow fibres. There was also a suggestion that the slow fibres may have acquired some of the characteristics of fast fibres.

These, and other studies have suggested that, with appropriate training, slow muscle fibres can become "faster" or more anaerobic, while fast fibres can become "slower" or more aerobic. However, the basic fibre type probably remains unchanged. It is, however, not certain whether muscle fibre type is determined at birth or whether it can be (or has been) changed by training in childhood or youth. In any case, it may not matter since the large variability in the type of fibre present in elite athletes' muscles suggests that other factors are at least as important in determining athletic success.

Effects of training on muscle

There are two types of training regimen to which muscles may be subjected. At one extreme, strength training uses heavy loads, briefly applied, and with a relatively small number of repetitions. The classic example of this type of training is weight lifting. On the other hand, endurance training uses quite light loads, which are applied continuously and for long periods of time. The classic example of this is long distance running. Of course, most athletes combine strength and endurance training sessions in various proportions.

strength training

One outcome of the manned space programme was the observation that in the absence of gravity the muscles which normally support the body atrophy or decrease in size, and become weak. Special training methods had to be devised to enable astronauts living in cramped spacecraft for long periods of time to maintain some of their muscle strength, and to stress their limbs sufficiently to minimise the loss of calcium from the skeleton (Ch. 10).

If a limb is exercised just once each day, the force produced during this exertion must be 20–30% of maximum effort for its muscles to maintain their condition. If the muscle is worked less than this, it becomes weaker. With more exertion, the muscle becomes stronger. Although this is a highly artificial situation, it illustrates the principles of strength training. Muscles which are asked to work hard become stronger, while those doing little work atrophy and weaken.

Strength training is accomplished by lifting weights, by contracting muscles against the elastic load of a heavy spring, or by straining against an immovable object such as a doorframe. There are any number of formal training regimens. In general they require something like ten repetitions of a task from as seldom as once each week to as often as twice each day. To be an effective form of training, the load chosen should require a force of at least 50% of the maximum capacity for that muscle group. Using a load requiring 100% of the muscle's capability may make it impossible to complete ten repetitions.

A strength training programme will usually include a series of tasks, each designed to train different muscle groups. In a varied programme, there is some evidence that little is gained if a task is repeated more often than three times each week, or if the loads used exceed 80% of the muscle's capacity to generate force. Heavier loads increase the likelihood of damage to muscles (see p. 242), tendons or joints. More frequent repetition will make it difficult for this damage to be repaired.

effectiveness of strength training
A ten-week weight training programme requiring forty minutes of work per day, twice weekly has been shown to achieve gains ranging from around 10% in grip and in biceps strength to nearly 30% in the force of the leg muscles. Muscle strength can be increased with surprisingly little effort. One study asked subjects to grip with maximum force for just one second every day. Within five weeks the average gain in grip strength was 33%.

The "trainability" of muscles varies widely. Basically, it depends on the previous use to which these muscles have been put. Thus, a weight lifting programme will have little effect on the leg strength of a hod-carrier, or on the grip strength of a brick-layer. On the other hand, remarkable results can be achieved if the subject is a sedentary desk worker.

The effectiveness of strength training depends on eating a diet with adequate protein. A protein intake of 1 gram per kilogram (g/kg/day) of body weight per day will support any realistic training programme. If the diet contains too little protein (less than 0.8 g/kg/day), muscle and strength development will not occur. At around 90 grams per day, the protein content of the typical European or American diet is more than adequate to support a high rate of muscle development. However, in some of the world's poorer countries, strength development is limited by diet, and during famine severe wasting is seen as muscle protein is used by the body for energy to maintain life.

Another factor is sex. Males are more "trainable" with respect to strength than females. This is due to the relative abundance of testosterone, the male sex hormone, in the two sexes (Fig. 2.11). Testosterone and synthetic hormones similar to it have been used by sportsmen and women to give them additional strength, and initially an advantage over their competitors (Ch. 9). There are serious dangers associated with using either natural or synthetic hormones to build strength, and if everyone uses such aids, there

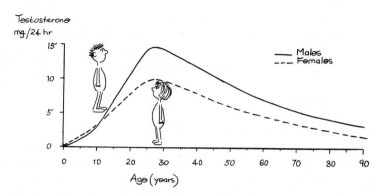

Fig. 2.11 *Testosterone production rises, reaching a peak at 25–30 years of age. After puberty, males produce nearly twice as much as females.*

is no advantage to be gained, only the disadvantage of permanent damage to health.

The ability to develop strength also depends on age. Following training, both males and females achieve the greatest gains when they are between 20 and 30 years of age. This is due to the amount of testosterone secreted. Its production increases steeply with age in both sexes, but reaches much higher values in males (Fig. 2.11). The peak testosterone production is achieved between the ages of 20 and 30, coinciding with the age at which strength training is most effective. Thereafter testosterone, and strength trainability, declines gradually.

what does strength training do?
Strength training is highly specific. Thus a true isometric regimen, or straining against an immovable object, produces greater improvement in maximal force than does a dynamic or isotonic regime of contracting against a movable weight. However, isotonic training improves the rate of force development (speed of contraction) far more than isometric training. Other characteristics of the training regimen are also important in determining the overall result.

The range of movement over which training occurs will result in the greatest development of strength within that range. If training uses slow limb movements, the result will be muscles which are

212271

strong only at slow speeds. Fast movement during training produces muscles capable of strength at both fast and slow contraction speeds. It is therefore important to consider the purpose to which the newly developed strength will be put.

factors responsible for increased strength
It is worth mentioning that a variety of psychological factors can play a role in strength performance. Thus, shouting during the test, drinking alcohol in advance, and hypnosis have all been shown to improve strength. However, the effects of shouting are most noticeable in the novice, almost vanishing in the seasoned competitor. Successful athletes in strength and power events probably enhance performance by concentration, achieving a state akin to self-hypnosis. The effects of skill must not be underestimated, even when related to an apparently simple task like weight lifting.

It has been shown that early in a strength training programme inprovements in performance are seen which are not accompanied by increases in muscle mass. One explanation of this is that muscles are normally inhibited from exerting their maximum effort, perhaps to protect the body from self-inflicted damage. In support of this, there is evidence that not all of the motor units which could participate in a movement are actually active during a maximum contraction. Accordingly, one aspect of strength training may be the removal of inhibition, allowing more of the muscle to participate in movement, thereby increasing strength.

The most important factor in the development of strength is muscle hypertrophy. When stressed, muscle fibres hypertrophy — they produce more contractile protein, becoming thicker and stronger. There is no evidence for a change in absolute strength — that is, strength relative to the muscle cross-section area. Increases in strength only occur in parallel with increases in the amount of muscle tissue present.

In some animal experiments, it has been suggested that training increases the number of muscle fibres. Normally adult muscle fibres do not divide to produce new daughter cells. Partially split muscle fibres have been seen in exercise trained animals whose muscles have hypertrophied. However, there is little evidence for either fibre splitting or for an increase in the number of muscle fibres in humans.

Athletes specialising in strength activities tend to have muscles composed predominantly of fast fibres. This has given rise to speculation that, with the right training, it may be possible to convert slow fibres into fast fibres. There is little evidence that this does happen, although it appears that slow fibres or intermediate types begin to behave more like fast fibres, that is, to improve their capacity for anaerobic metabolism. However, the effects of training are quite specific. Strength training mainly causes hypertrophy in the fast fibres which tend to be used during this type of work. So the total mass of fast fibres, if not their number, does increase, while there is far less change in the mass (or number) of slow fibres in the same muscle.

changes in metabolism in strength training

Strength training gives the body very little metabolic stimulation. This is because the total amount of work accomplished during weight lifting (for example) is small. Although the weights may represent a very heavy load, this load is only moved a short distance, and borne very briefly. So during a one hour session, not much more than 5 minutes might be spent in actual lifting. The

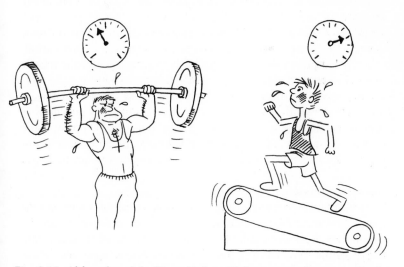

Fig. 2.12 Although weight lifters look as if they are working very hard indeed, their energy expenditure during training is considerably less than that of an endurance runner. Because of this, weight training has little effect on the performance of the heart.

heart rate, typically, will average only 130 beats per minute, and oxygen consumption may be no more than three times the resting value. Few strength training regimes even double the metabolic rate of walking on the level! This level of work provides little stimulation to the metabolic processes, and does not tax the cardiovascular system's ability to deliver oxygen.

However, the cardiovascular system is altered by strength training. During powerful muscle contraction, major arteries passing through the working muscles are obstructed, raising the blood pressure — often dramatically. The heart muscle responds by becoming thicker and stronger. Often, the ventricles even become smaller in volume. This helps them to continue pumping blood against the high arterial pressures which occur during isometric muscle contraction.

A second response is a modest increase in the density of blood capillaries within the muscle. Although much of the work during isometric contraction is anaerobic, a great deal of lactic acid is produced, and the blood flow must increase to keep the tissue from becoming too acid.

Within muscle fibres, strength training causes no increase in the numbers of mitochondria, where the aerobic production of ATP takes place (see Ch. 3). By increasing the amount of contractile machinery (muscle mass) served by the existing mitochondria, training for power may even diminish endurance. Since the body mass also rises, the amount of work associated with a particular activity increases, further taxing endurance. In support of this, it has been shown that when a power athlete stops training, his/her aerobic capacity and endurance actually improve. The other side of the coin is that undertaking both strength and endurance training at the same time interferes with strength development.

electrical stimulation
To rehabilitate people recovering from wasting following injury, temporary paralysis, or surgery, muscles may be activated by stimulation with electrical currents applied to the skin. It is therefore possible to "exercise" muscles whose nerves have been damaged, or in people who are not able to exercise.

Ever on the lookout for new techniques to improve performance, electrical muscle stimulation has been used in an attempt to increase strength and speed. Unfortunately, improvements in performance are largely limited to the specific movements attempted in training. Probably because electrical stimulation of the muscle surface produces crude contractions which do not mimic movement, there is no evidence of improvement in strength or speed. Of course, in patients suffering from wasting due to prolonged immobilisation (after wearing a cast or other prosthesis, or waiting for the regeneration of a damaged nerve) this technique is effective in rebuilding strength.

Electrical stimulation is used in "health studios" where it is claimed that the technique will help shed fat. Using this technique, a person can have their muscles exercised without thinking about it, perhaps while reading a book or basking in the glow of a sunlamp. The author doubts that it actually works, since fairly heroic energy expenditure is required to produce weight loss (p. 239). Applying an electrical current to the skin stimulates sense organs located there. The amount of stimulation which may be applied is thus limited by the pain and discomfort this causes, and also by the potential damage which may be caused if the disorganised muscle contractions are too powerful.

Endurance training

Endurance training is accomplished by selecting a relatively light work load, carrying this out regularly, and for long periods of time. Clearly, the work load cannot be too hard, or it will be impossible to sustain for the time necessary to achieve an endurance training effect. On the other hand, it must be of sufficient intensity to be effective. Initially, a chosen work load might be around 50% of the VO_{2max}. In time, as training proceeds, the work intensity may be increased to 80% of VO_{2max} or even higher.

A programme of endurance training almost always centres on the leg muscles. These muscles normally have a large proportion of slow muscle fibres and are capable of reasonable endurance performance even without training. Typical endurance activities include running, bicycling, swimming, and cross-country skiing.

The effects of strength training are virtually confined to muscle, making improvements quite simple to assess. During endurance training, many of the observed effects are related to the considerable and prolonged increase in metabolic rate which is experienced.

Thus, the aerobic capability of muscle is improved (Ch. 3), as are the physiological systems involved in the supply of oxygen and removal of carbon dioxide (Ch. 5 & 6), and heat (Ch. 7). This makes it difficult to measure and assess the changes occurring within muscle on their own. In general, there is little effect on muscle strength.

Within the muscle, two major changes can be seen. First, the number of mitochondria increases. These are the small organs within the cells where oxygen is consumed and ATP is generated. A muscle's ability to consume oxygen is partly determined by the number of mitochondria it possesses. It is not entirely certain what causes the number of mitochondria to increase, but it may be due to the local reduction in oxygen partial pressure which occurs during aerobic exercise. Mitochondrial numbers are also high in residents of high altitude who are exposed to a reduced oxygen pressure.

In parallel with the increase in numbers of mitochondria, there is an increase in the density of capillaries and other small blood vessels within the body of the muscle. Capillaries and mitochondria appear to proliferate together so that muscles with large numbers of mitochondria always have an abundance of capillaries. As with mitochondria, the stimuli which cause capillaries to grow are not well understood. A low oxygen environment encourages capillary growth. A high rate of blood flow within a tissue also stimulates capillary growth, possibly due to turbulent blood flow, or to the increased blood pressure within the capillaries. Another stimulant of capillary growth is the accumulation of metabolic wastes.

During endurance training, the working muscles are exposed to all three factors — low oxygen, a high rate of blood flow, and the accumulation of metabolic wastes — for relatively long periods of time, and their high density network of capillaries may be the result.

CHAPTER THREE

Metabolism

To extract useful work from fuels, man-made machines oxidise or burn them at high temperature. The resulting heat is then used to produce motion and hence power. The efficiency of such machines is determined by the temperature at which combustion occurs, which in turn is limited to around 800°C by the materials which are used to construct and lubricate them, materials which would melt or burn if they became too hot. Unless very high combustion temperatures are achieved using special heat resistant alloys or even ceramics, only 40% of the chemical energy contained in a fuel can be realised as external work. This means that at least 60% of the energy in a fuel is wasted as heat.

Metabolism is a remarkable process which routinely equals the efficiency of many machines, without violent combustion, and at a relatively cool (body) temperature. Chemical energy is obtained from foodstuffs in gradual stages. At each stage energy is transferred to and stored in special high energy compounds, from which it can be readily released when required. The energy is stored by attaching phosphate to molecules of adenosine or creatine. This forms adenosine tri-phosphate or ATP (adenosine with three phosphates attached), and phosphocreatine or PCr (creatine with one attached phosphate). When needed, the energy is then retrieved by splitting phosphate away from the ATP or PCr.

The efficiency of oxidative phosphorylation (the process of obtaining the energy to attach phosphate to adenosine) is 65% (0.65). Using the stored energy of ATP by converting it into mechanical work is accomplished at an efficiency of 41% (0.41). Hence, the expected efficiency of converting food into motion is $0.65 \times 0.41 = 0.27$, or 27%. Comparing the actual amount of food energy required to produce a measured work output, the body usually operates at an efficiency of 15–20%, only rarely achieving 25%. The discrepancy exists because auxiliary systems must be powered too: breathing, the cardiovascular system, excretion of wastes, the repair of cells, etc. These processes operate

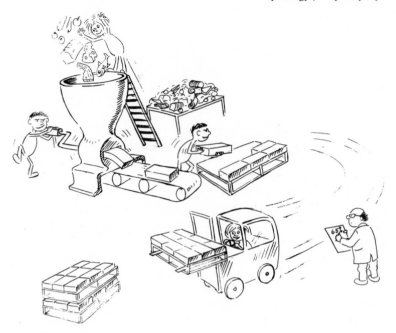

Fig. 3.1 Our energy is derived from the food we eat. We store energy in various forms (see Fig. 3.8). We convert food energy into ATP with an efficiency of 65%

continuously, consuming energy but producing no output work. As work output increases, the proportion of the metabolic rate devoted to these auxiliary systems diminishes and efficiency rises towards the theoretical maximum of 27%.*

Clearly most of the energy contained in food is not used for mechanical work. This "wasted energy" appears as heat. Heat production is often desirable because it maintains the body temperature in a cool environment. Indeed, much of the time the

---

* Actually, under carefully chosen conditions of speed and load, somewhat greater efficiencies can be realised by using the kinetic energy of motion and the elastic energy stored in flexing bones and in stretched muscles & tendons. Thus, in running, part of the energy absorbed during a landing can be retrieved when taking off for the next step. It is likely that athletes and trainers take advantage of this, probably without realising that they are doing so. The body's flexibility and elasticity also protects it from damage.

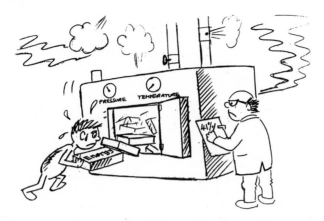

Fig. 3.2 We "burn" or use energy (as ATP) with an efficiency of 41%. Together with the 65% efficiency of forming ATP, overall only 27% of our food energy yields some form of useful work.

body's heat production is inadequate, and heat from external sources is eagerly sought. However, during hard work a great deal of heat must be lost. Sometimes, when the environmental temperature is high, heat loss is a problem (see Ch. 7). Food energy is also used to break down and rebuild tissue, to produce hormones and digestive juices, or is simply lost as hair, skin, or fingernails, etc.

Energy sources and ATP

The chemical energy of ATP is used to power all of the activities of the body: movement of muscles, formation of secretions, transmission of nerve impulses, manufacture and repair of tissues, etc. Stored ATP is broken down to adenosine di-phosphate (ADP) and the energy liberated is used to power chemical reactions. ADP is then converted back into ATP to maintain the stores (Equation 1). Although the body's store of ATP is very small (enough to satisfy the body's requirements for 1–2 minutes at rest), the total weight of ATP which is turned over (broken down and regenerated) each day is approximately equal to the entire body weight!

ATP is the "common currency" of the body. All of the body's fuels are converted into ATP before being used, and their energy content is stored in ATP. The main such fuels are carbohydrate (eg

Equation 1

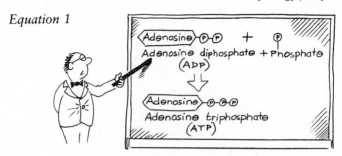

starch) and fat. Although protein is also used, it normally contributes around 10% to the total energy supply. These substances are "burned", in the presence of oxygen, at body temperature, to yield water, carbon dioxide, and ATP.

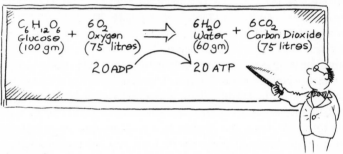

Equation 2

All chemical reactions take place between specific numbers of molecules. Since the weights of the molecules are known, the quantities of the various materials taking part in a reaction can be expressed in terms which we can understand. Let us take glucose and palmitic acid as representative carbohydrate and fat respectively, and consider the metabolism of 100 grams of each in the body (Equations 2 & 3).

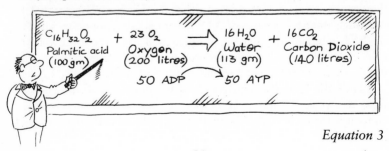

Equation 3

The Respiratory Exchange Ratio (R), is the ratio of CO_2 produced and O_2 used. When the body metabolises carbohydrate (or protein), the volume of carbon dioxide lost is equal to the volume of oxygen taken up (equations above) and R = 1. For a pure fat diet, R = 140/200 = 0.7. Typically R is 0.85 reflecting our "western" diet in which 40−45% of the energy comes from fat. R can be used as an index of the proportion of fat and carbohydrate being oxidised at any time.

A carbohydrate molecule contains far more oxygen (it starts out partly oxidised) than a similar weight of fat. Therefore, dietary fats yield 2.5 times as much energy (ATP) on oxidation as would an equal weight of carbohydrate. Moreover, since protein and carbohydrate based foods (meat, rice, etc) tend to be watery, while fatty foods (nuts, cheese, etc) usually contain little water, the energy content of fatty foods is normally considerably more than 2.5 times that of starchy foods. Thus butter yields nearly four times as much energy as an equal weight of bread, and six times more than the same weight of boiled rice.

Although the energy from foodstuffs must be converted into ATP before powering the body's systems, energy intake or expenditure is not expressed in units of ATP. Instead, energy intake is expressed as kilocalories (kcal), or the more modern unit kilojoules (kJ), per day (1 kcal = 4.2 kJ). This can be estimated by weighing and recording the daily food consumption, and then using tables which list the energy content of the foods eaten.

Energy expenditure can be expressed in units of work such as kilojoules, or in units of power (work rate) such as Watts (Joules/second). Since the energy expenditure is generally measured indirectly, by recording the rate of oxygen consumption, energy expenditure may also be expressed in terms of oxygen, and converted into units of work or power:

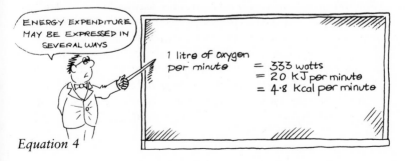

ENERGY EXPENDITURE MAY BE EXPRESSED IN SEVERAL WAYS

1 litre of oxygen per minute
= 333 watts
= 20 kJ per minute
= 4·8 Kcal per minute

Equation 4

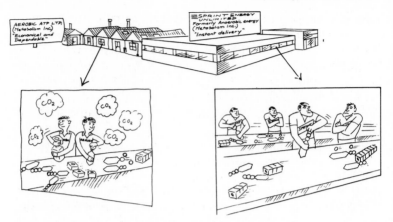

Fig. 3.3 Every cell has within itself two metabolic factories producing ATP: the first operates anaerobically (without oxygen) and can work very fast; the second works aerobically and more slowly. The two are linked because the end product of the first is used by the second.

Work rate and oxygen consumption

As the work rate increases, the rate of fuel oxidation must rise to supply the ATP (energy) required for muscle contraction. The rate at which oxygen is used by a cell is probably controlled by the amount of ADP present. If ATP is being used rapidly, the concentration of ADP rises and oxygen utilisation is stimulated to re-attach phosphates back onto ADP, converting it into ATP. In due course, high rates of work will require an increased intake of food to prevent depletion of energy stores, and weight loss.

Once the work rate has increased to about 60% of an individual's maximum, shortages of oxygen begin to occur and anaerobic metabolism is stimulated. This process regenerates ATP without using oxygen, but gives rise to the byproduct, lactic acid. Using anaerobic metabolism, work rates corresponding to over 300% of the maximum oxygen consumption may be achieved, although accumulation of lactic acid (see Oxygen Debt, p. 43) strictly limits the time that this rate of work can be maintained.

The following table illustrates the relationship between work output and oxygen consumption for a "standard" 70 kg (11 st) man:

Table 3.1 *The energy cost of work*

Work (70 kg man)	Oxygen consumption (ml/min)	Energy expenditure (watts)	(kcal/min)	(kJ/min)
Rest	250	85	1.2	5.0
Moderate work	1,000	333	4.8	20.1
Hard work	2,000	667	9.6	40.2
Maximal work	4,000	1,333	19.2	80.4

where:
Moderate work — can be sustained daily, for a full working day,
Hard work — can be sustained for a full day by the physically fit, but then only for a few days,
Maximal work — is exhausting within a short time.

It is worth emphasising that the heat production (energy expenditure) of a hard working person is equivalent to one bar of an

Table 3.2

Activity	Time (hr)	Oxygen consumption (ml/min)	(l/day)	Energy equivalent (kcal/day)	(kJ/day)
Basal rate	24	250	360	1,700	7,100
+ extra for:					
Office work	8	200	96	460	1,925
Sitting (home)	6	75	18	90	375
Eating	1.5	100	9	45	190
Walking	0.5	800	24	115	480
Sedentary total			507	2,400	10,000
Run @ 10 mph	1.0	3,500	230	1,100	4,600
Active total			737	3,500	14,600

electric fire. It is thus not unexpected that running at 7.5 mph (twice walking speed or eight minute miles) or playing a brisk game of squash, both equivalent to an energy expenditure of 1000 Watts, cause one to become very hot, very rapidly (Ch. 7).

energy economy during a day
Surprisingly, except for people who train for over an hour each day, energy expenditure during exercise contributes little to the daily energy requirement.

In the example in Table 3.2 it is clear that, despite a long and energetic training regime, the basal metabolic rate still accounts for most of the day's energy expenditure. It is easy to see why the modest levels of exercise achieved by most people who wish to lose weight are rarely effective.

where is the energy used?
The body is not homogeneous. Its various tissues and organs have very different functions and widely differing energy requirements.

Table 3.3 *Components of the metabolic rate of a 70 kg man*

Organ	Weight (kg)	Oxygen consumption (ml/min)		% of resting rate	
		Rest	Max.	Rest	Max.
Brain	1.4	47	47	19	1
Heart	0.3	17	1,000	7	25
Kidneys	0.3	26	20	10	1
Liver	1.6	67	100?	27	3
Muscle	30.0	45	2,800	18	70
Other	35.0	48	35	19	1
Total	70.0	250	4,000	100	100

Some 40–50% of the body's weight is muscle, although it accounts for less than 20% of the resting metabolic rate. In exercise, muscle energy requirement increases by over 50 times. The brain's metabolic rate is high considering its relatively small size (about 5% of the body's muscle mass). Its requirements and those of most other tissues are relatively unaffected by physical activity. In maximum activity, the metabolic rates of skeletal muscle and heart muscle dwarf the requirements of the rest of the body.

How is energy stored in the body?

The body stores several forms of energy. The largest store is fat, of which even lean people have enough to supply their needs for over thirty days. In fact, it is not possible to use all of the fat reserves in starvation because the supply of various other substances run short, threatening health and survival.

Carbohydrate is mainly stored as glycogen ("animal starch"), of which there is enough for about twelve hours of sedentary activity. Glycogen is a polymer of glucose and its use allows sugar to be stored in a compact form. In addition, a small amount (about twenty minutes worth) of glucose is stored in the extracellular fluid (the fluid surrounding cells). Although only a small amount is stored, it is important because a steady concentration of glucose is maintained, and this is delivered by the blood supply to all the tissues in the body.

Table 3.4 *The body's energy inventory*

	Amount	*Theoretical endurance*	
		At rest	*Hard work*
Adenosine tri-phosphate (ATP)	90 g.	1–2 mins	1–2 secs
Creatine phosphate (PCr)	120 g.	4–6 mins	10 secs
Glycogen	350 g.	12 hrs	40–60 mins
Fat*	3–25+ kg	30+ days	no limit
Protein (can use 30–40%)	12–14 kg	8–10 days	no limit

* Variable — depends on degree of obesity.

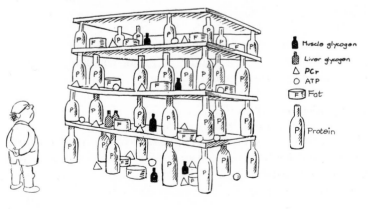

Protein can also supply energy. However, little protein is used unless the diet contains a surplus. No "official" stores of protein are kept for energy. Rather, muscle and other protein is depleted when usual energy supplies run short. Using this protein progressively deprives muscles of their contractile mechanism, weakening the body. However, the body must rely on protein in starvation (and crash diets) when certain amino acids are used to generate the glucose fuel vital to some tissues (mainly the brain) which are unable to use fat.

All tissues have a store of ATP to power activity instantly. In theory, the store of ATP in the body would supply two minutes of resting metabolic activity. However, ATP is never depleted by resting tissues, and only minimally depleted in moderate activity. Maximally active muscle is able to use almost half of its stored ATP to give an endurance of just one or two seconds.

Backing up ATP is phosphocreatine (PCr, see p. 31) whose energy can be used to regenerate ATP very quickly. The body has stores of PCr containing enough energy for four to six minutes of resting metabolism, but again, neither resting nor moderately active tissues actually deplete PCr. It is not certain how much depletion of a muscle's PCr stores is possible, even in vigorous activity, but it appears that ATP and PCr together can support 10–13 seconds of maximal work.

Theoretically, the body contains enough high energy phosphate compounds (ATP and PCr) to survive for 6–7 minutes at rest without oxygen. However, one cannot actually live that long without oxygen. Individual tissues store variable amounts of high energy phosphates. Without oxygen, tissues like the brain run short of energy and begin to die within two to three minutes. On the other hand, blood supplies to skin, muscle, or the intestine can be interrupted for many minutes without harm. Thus, a tourniquet could be applied to a limb for up to thirty minutes (but don't try this!) before causing serious damage.

where is energy stored?
There are three sites for energy storage in the body: (i) individual cells have their own stores of ATP, PCr, glycogen, and fat; (ii) the liver is a central store of glycogen; and (iii) various depots around the body store fats.

Each cell has a store of ATP and PCr. This ensures that any energy requiring activity — muscular contraction, structural repair, or hormone secretion — can begin instantly if required.

Glycogen is also stored locally, and the stimulation of its use by metabolism depends upon changes in the ratio of ADP to ATP (only trivial depletion of ATP occurs at all but the highest work loads). Glycogen is found in all cells, with muscle and liver having particularly generous stores. In a 70 kg man, approximately 30 kg of muscle contain 245 g of glycogen. Although the human liver weighs less than 2 kg, it contains 110 g, or nearly seven times the glycogen found in a similar weight of muscle. When required the liver breaks down its glycogen producing glucose, which is transported in the blood to supply other tissues.

The largest "official" energy store is fat. Various depots of fat are located around the body, under the skin, around the kidneys and around the heart. Fat must be liberated or mobilised from these depots and brought to working tissues by the bloodstream. This cannot be done rapidly, so fat only becomes a useful source of energy after 15–20 minutes of exercise (below). Abundant stores of fat offer a person no endurance advantage. Obese individuals have trouble using fat as fuel at all (Ch. 10). In any case, even a lean person weighing just 50 kg has at least 2 kg of stored fat. This is ample for 20 hours of hard work! Only long distance swimmers make use of fat stores, but for insulation and buoyancy, not energy.

The total weight of protein in the body is large, and represents a huge energy store. Realistically, less than 20 per cent of this energy can be made available without damage to the body. This is enough to ensure that endurance is never limited by protein energy stores. However, in starvation as much as 40 per cent (depending on circumstances) of the body's protein may be sacrificed to sustain life. After 20–30 days of starvation, permanent damage through tissue wasting may occur. (On the other hand, well-upholstered volunteers have endured up to six months of fasting under medical supervision without harm!)

how do we begin to use energy?
When activity begins, stored ATP is used during the initial seconds of activity. The rising concentration of ADP (and other products

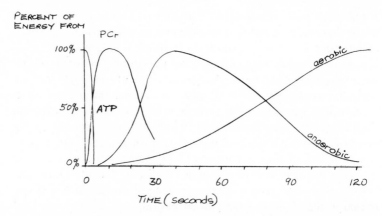

Fig. 3.5 In the first few seconds of moderate work (less than half of VO_{2MAX}), all energy is obtained anaerobically. Within thirty seconds aerobic processes have begun to supply ATP. By two minutes, anaerobic metabolism has been run down to provide about 5% of requirements. At moderate work loads most of the energy is supplied aerobically. However, no matter how light the work some energy always comes from anaerobic metabolism.

of ATP breakdown*) stimulates metabolism. There is very little ADP in resting muscle, and a small depletion of ATP is amplified into a large increase in the concentration of ADP, which becomes a sensitive trigger for metabolism. At first, ATP is regenerated from PCr, which donates its high energy phosphate to ADP. In the first ten seconds of activity, most of the energy used is supplied by stored PCr (Fig. 3.5).

By thirty seconds, glucose becomes the major source of energy to regenerate ATP from ADP and phosphate. The first step in glucose metabolism, glycolysis, is anaerobic (requires no oxygen). This step is very fast, but yields only two ATPs per molecule of glucose used and creates lactic acid which can accumulate (see below). The next step is aerobic (requires oxygen). This is slower, but yields a massive thirty-four ATPs per molecule of glucose.

---

* AMP (adenosine monophosphate) is probably also formed, by stripping off a second high energy phosphate. Rising AMP concentration may also play a role in stimulating metabolism.

Aerobic metabolism has begun by thirty seconds, and takes over much (over 95%) of the body's energy supply within two minutes.

Breathing begins to respond to activity only after a delay of half a minute. If you sprint up three flights of stairs and then sit down, your breathing will accelerate perhaps ten seconds after you have stopped moving. It takes some sixty seconds for the body to start to consume oxygen. This is due to the delay in switching on aerobic metabolism (Fig. 3.5). The continued high rate of respiration after exercise has stopped has been called an "oxygen debt".

Oxygen debt

During physical activity, breathing effort and oxygen consumption rise. However, both lag behind work output at the start of exercise (above), and continue above the resting level for some time after activity stops. During the first two minutes, less oxygen is taken up by the body than is required for the work load. After exercise stops, oxygen consumption remains high for some time, and this deficit or oxygen debt is said to be "paid back".

An oxygen debt does appear to accumulate during hard exercise, and for many years it was thought that the elevated rate of oxygen consumption which followed afterwards "pays this back". It is now known that little of the extra oxygen consumed post-exercise actually pays off the energy debt. For this reason, the expression "oxygen debt" is not strictly correct, but it is vivid and will be used here.

If an individual works at a load requiring 2.5 litres of oxygen for four minutes a total of ten litres of oxygen will be needed. Although the person may be capable of aerobic work at that level of effort, in fact much of this work load will actually be performed anaerobically (Fig. 3.6). This is because oxygen uptake does not reach the 2.5 litre per minute mark until two minutes have passed and some four litres of oxygen (above the normal resting intake) are absorbed during the post-exercise recovery period.

Imagine the same individual engaged in a sprint run requiring 20 litres of oxygen per minute and lasting 0.5 minute (Fig. 3.6). Now, the oxygen uptake only has time to reach one litre per minute by the time activity stops, leaving most of the oxygen cost to be made up during the post-exercise rest period. The oxygen debt has two parts, a "fast" and a "slow" component.

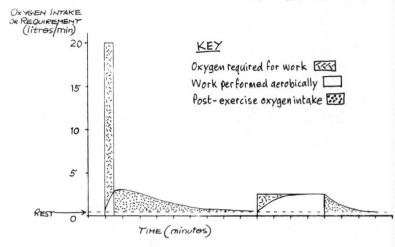

Fig. 3.6

fast component

The fast component of oxygen debt is the brief increase in metabolic rate required to recycle the ADP to ATP and to regenerate the PCr depleted during activity. Some ADP must accumulate however gentle the activity, because a change in its concentration is required to stimulate metabolism. The post-exercise conversion of ADP to ATP and restoration of PCr is very quick, and probably complete in less than one minute (making it hard to study with precision). The slow component is partly due to the accumulation of lactic acid.

slow component (lactic acid)

At work loads requiring more than half of an individual's maximum oxygen intake, lactic acid begins to appear in the blood. This is because glucose, a six carbon atom molecule, is metabolised in two stages (Fig. 3.7). First, there is a fast anaerobic step which takes place in the fluid of the cell. This splits glucose in half, to yield two ATPs and two pyruvates (a three carbon atom precursor of lactic acid). This is followed by an aerobic step which uses the pyruvate and yields thirty-four ATPs plus carbon dioxide (Equation 2). This is carried out in special cell structures called the

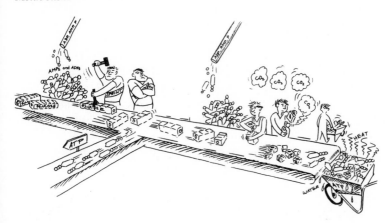

Fig. 3.7

mitochondria. Although the second step yields far more energy than the first, it is also slower. So when the work load is high and ADP begins to accumulate, stimulation of the fast anaerobic step generates more pyruvic acid than the slow aerobic step can use (Fig. 3.8). Pyruvate accumulates within the cell and is converted to

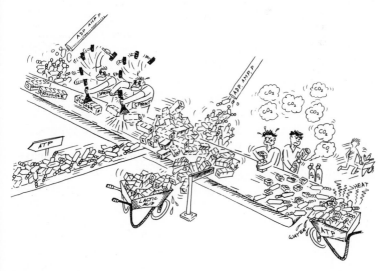

Fig. 3.8

lactic acid* by taking up hydrogen ions (which are abundant during exercise).

Lactic acid accumulation within a tissue impairs its ability to carry out anaerobic metabolism, and its ability to use ATP as well. Fortunately, lactic acid is exported from the muscle and is efficiently removed by the circulation. The liver and the heart take lactic acid out of the blood and use it in their own aerobic metabolism. However, if too much is produced, lactic acid begins to accumulate in the blood, eventually inhibiting metabolism and activity. This is one reason why high rates of activity are rapidly fatiguing.

After exercise stops, lactic acid must be cleared from the blood. This is accomplished partly by reversing glycolysis — glucose and glycogen can be rebuilt from lactic acid. This process requires energy and oxygen, giving rise to a period of increased oxygen consumption following exercise. Of course, activity uses glycogen, and recovery cannot be said to be complete until these stores are entirely replenished, normally only after a meal.

slow component (miscellaneous)

Lactic acid is also used aerobically in the cell to generate ATP. The greater part of the accumulated lactic acid is dealt with in this manner. The remainder of the slow component of oxygen debt is due to an elevated metabolic rate arising from several circumstances.

The high body temperature at the end of exercise has the effect of increasing both the metabolic rate and the oxygen consumption. Since it may take over ten minutes to cool down, the metabolic rate will remain elevated that long. The various hormones such as adrenaline, noradrenaline, growth hormone, and others released during activity also persist in the blood, and continue to stimulate metabolism for some time after activity stops.

Cardiac output too remains high after exercise, probably partly due to the need to dissipate heat, and partly due to the influence of the lactic acid still present in the blood, both of which dilate vascular beds, increasing the demand for blood flow.

---

* In the blood, lactic acid is rapidly converted by buffering into sodium lactate, which most scientists simply call "lactate". However, the term lactic acid is used here because it is more familiar.

summary

To illustrate the importance of the oxygen debt in relation to the energy demands of exercise, imagine an individual running in a series of races. In a 100m sprint (10 seconds), 85% of the energy is supplied by anaerobic processes. In an 800m run (105 seconds), 50% of the energy is anaerobic in origin. A 3000m run (8 minutes) is only 15% dependent on anaerobic metabolism. Finally, a marathon (2.5 hr) is 99% aerobic.

Some of the extra oxygen consumed post-exercise is genuinely a repaid "oxygen debt" or "energy debt". This portion is the regeneration of ATP stores, the clearing of accumulated lactic acid, and the rebuilding of glycogen stores. However, much is simply due to an elevated metabolic rate which persists until the body temperature, hormones, accumulated wastes, and energy stores all return to normal.

Tests or indices of physical fitness

Tests of physical fitness either test the body's ability to clear its oxygen debt and return to rest after a period of work, or measure the degree to which metabolic processes may be stimulated by set work loads.

resting heart rate

Resting heart rate is the simplest (and crudest) index of physical fitness. Fit individuals tend to have far slower heart rates than sedentary people. In the sedentary population the heart rate averages about 70 beats per minute. The heart rates of endurance athletes are usually less than 50 beats per minute, and occasionally less than 40.

heart rate during post-exercise recovery

The heart rate increases rapidly during exercise from 60–70 beats per minute to a maximum of 180–220 per minute (see Ch. 6). After the completion of a work load, the heart rate gradually recovers to its resting value. The simplest test of physical fitness is based on the speed of this recovery. An athlete's heart rate will return to its resting value faster than that of a sedentary individual.

With this test the choice of work load raises a problem. A harder work load stimulates the heart rate more and creates a longer lasting oxygen debt. This gives rise to a longer, slower recovery than a light load. Since larger people are usually stronger and capable of higher work loads than smaller people, if everyone is tested at the same load, larger individuals would tend to recover faster and thus appear more fit.

If a cycle ergometer can be used for the test, the work load could be set according to the subject's weight with, say, two Watts output per kilogram of body weight. In a step test, the subject steps up and down one or two steps for two minutes at thirty repetitions per minute. This is simple, cheap, and since the subject works against their own weight, it compensates for differences in body bulk. However, the step test uses a fixed height step, and may be inappropriate for particularly short or tall subjects.) Following such a test, a sedentary person recovers to resting heart rate in 10–15 minutes, an athlete in two to three minutes.

maximum oxygen uptake (VO_{2MAX})
The development of the ability to use oxygen at a high rate used to be a leading aim of a training programme. Indeed, training (increasing one's habitual level of activity) does influence the ability to use oxygen — hence the ability to do work. One characteristic of competitive endurance athletes is that they often have very high values of VO_{2MAX}. Thus, where a typical young male might be able to use three to four litres of oxygen per minute, a champion distance runner or cyclist would be capable of five to seven litres per minute. It was logical to believe that training increased the VO_{2MAX}, and that this was a principal means of achieving improvements in performance.

The VO_{2MAX} test is performed by having the subject work continuously, on a treadmill or a stationary cycle, against a series of increasing work loads. Eventually, a point is reached at which further increases in load fail to increase the oxygen consumption (Fig. 3.9), the extra work being performed anaerobically. The oxygen consumption at this point is the VO_{2MAX}. Exhaustion occurs quickly near the VO_{2MAX}, and the test is always performed with some idea what the VO_{2MAX} value is so that no more than six ascending work loads (15–20 minutes of total exercise) are required. It is worth noting that the volume of air moved by the respiratory system begins to increase very steeply when anaerobic metabolism begins in earnest (Ch. 4).

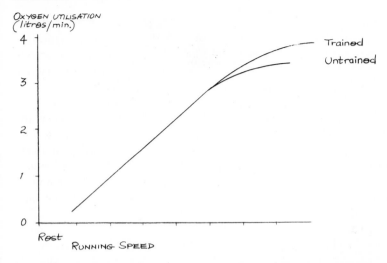

Fig. 3.9 As speed increases, the oxygen consumption rises steadily. Eventually, a further rise in speed fails to increase oxygen consumption. This oxygen consumption is the VO_{2MAX}. The extra speed is powered by anaerobic metabolism and cannot be sustained for long. Training increases VO_{2MAX} slightly (Fig. 3.14).

VO_{2MAX} is cumbersome to measure and the test is not often performed. The method used will depend on what one seeks to achieve. For example, in a student practical class, each work load is maintained for two to three minutes to allow the subject's responses to stabilise. The oxygen consumption and heart rate are either monitored continuously, or measured during the final minute of each work load, the test taking 15–20 minutes. The result of such a test is a series of values illustrating oxygen consumption (heart rate is usually also measured) at various work loads. Ideally, the oxygen consumption should not change between the two final work loads, establishing the VO_{2MAX}.

A variant on this method is the discontinuous test. Here the subject works for five minutes, rests for five minutes and works another five minutes at a higher load. This sequence is repeated as required until the test is complete. The discontinuous test would be used for untrained individuals whose endurance is too limited to tolerate twenty minutes of continuous testing.

If a well trained athlete is being tested, perhaps for research purposes, his/her VO_{2MAX} may already be known from previous tests. In this case, a test might be carried out at just two loads — one at the point of a pre-determined VO_{2MAX}, and a second higher load. Here, one would expect to see no change in oxygen consumption between the two loads, establishing the VO_{2MAX} as above, but saving time by omitting the sub-maximal series.

There is little difference in the measured VO_{2MAX} using the continuous or discontinuous procedures, or in the short test used by researchers. A test carried out on a treadmill generally gives slightly higher values than on a stationary cycle, probably because more muscles are involved in running (and supporting one's body weight) than in cycling.

onset of blood lactate accumulation (OBLA) test
The ability to perform aerobic work is very different from the VO_{2MAX} and may be tested. This is done by giving subjects consecutive increases in work load (4–5 minutes at each level) on a treadmill or bicycle ergometer while measuring their oxygen consumption and heart rate. Blood samples are taken at the end of each work load and analysed for lactic acid. When the blood lactic acid concentration reaches an accepted value (usually 4 millimols per litre), this is said to be the point of lactate accumulation or OBLA (Fig. 3.10). This is similar to the continuous VO_{2MAX} test, except that there is no need to go to very high work rates, and fatigue is less of a problem. The work load at which lactic acid begins to accumulate in blood is called the anaerobic threshold.

The work load, heart rate and oxygen consumption at OBLA are noted, and are the result of the test. Once the athlete is aware of his/her heart rate at OBLA, this information can be used to establish a training regime. However, most trained athletes are able to sense their anaerobic threshold fairly accurately without ever being tested, and rarely work at either a higher or lower level for long.

A high work load or oxygen consumption (high % of VO_{2MAX}) at OBLA means that the individual can perform at a high level without accumulating lactic acid. Since lactic acid accumulation is one of the factors which limits the ability to continue, OBLA or anaerobic threshold is an index of the useful endurance speed.

In untrained individuals, the anaerobic threshold typically occurs at 50–60% of the maximum oxygen consumption. With

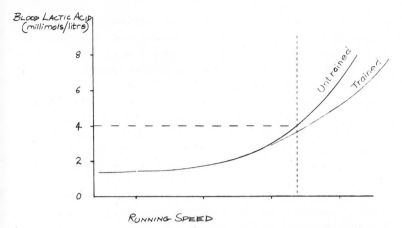

Fig. 3.10 At slow speeds, the lactic acid concentration in the blood remains low and constant. As speed increases, the anaerobic threshold is approached, and lactic acid rises steeply. Training reduces lactic acid production and shifts the anaerobic threshold to the right; lack of training does the reverse.

endurance training, this may rise to 85% of VO_{2MAX}, or even higher (Fig. 3.14). Individuals with a high anaerobic threshold are likely to do well in athletic events requiring endurance. That said, a good anaerobic threshold is no guarantee of a champion — although OBLA is a better guide than is the VO_{2MAX}.

Children behave differently to adults. Even at high work loads, they produce little lactic acid. A number of workers have reported that even when working at 70–80% of VO_{2MAX} children still do not exceed two millimols per litre of lactic acid. The muscles of children may be relatively deficient in the enzymes of glycolysis. It is not clear what effect this has on sprint performance, or on aerobic performance and endurance. It has been suggested that this may be a protective mechanism, reducing the peak rate of anaerobic work that children can produce, thereby preventing damage to their incompletely calcified skeleton.

the Wingate test for anaerobic power

The Wingate test has the subject perform work at a very high (sprint) rate for a brief period. The purpose of the test is to measure the maximum power output over thirty seconds. The test is kept short so that the contribution of aerobic metabolism to performance will be zero or very small. Consequently, it is a measure of the ability to perform glycolysis or anaerobic metabolism in the muscle groups tested.

Initially, the subject warms up on the bicycle ergometer for several minutes at a work load which causes the heart rate to reach 150 beats per minute. Then, following a 3–4 minute rest, the test begins. The subject initially accelerates the ergometer's flywheel, pedalling at 100 cycles per minute with no load. When this speed has been reached, the load is applied and the subject continues pedalling as fast as possible, for thirty seconds. The work performed is measured by counting the wheel revolutions and multiplying by the load applied.

Reasonably fit young men can produce peak outputs of 800–1200 Watts, declining to 600–800 Watts after thirty seconds. Women achieve 70% of these values. The peak power, which normally occurs during the first five seconds, is considered to come mainly from stored ATP. The lowest power, during the last five seconds, is compared to the peak to give the rate of decline or fatigue rate. Thus, if peak power is 900 Watts and lowest power is 500 Watts, the decline is (900−500)/900 × 100 = 44% — that is the lowest power is only 44% of the peak output. Power decline ranges from 95% to 30% or lower. Endurance runners and seden-

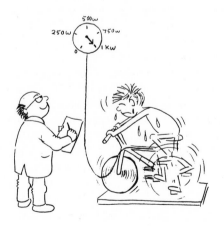

Fig. 3.11

tary people tend to have low maximum power and high rates of decline in this test, while sprinters and football players have a high anaerobic power, which is also well maintained.

An alternative (and cheaper) test of anaerobic power is based on the speed of stair climbing. The subject is allowed a number of stairs for acceleration, and his/her speed is measured by placing pressure sensitive pads on two of the stair treads which start and stop a clock. The work is done lifting the body over the measured height of stairs and the power output or rate of work is calculated by the speed at which this is done. This test is limited to testing the peak anaerobic power output, and gives no indication of anaerobic endurance.

Improving metabolic performance

sources of energy in prolonged moderate exercise
At the start of exercise, metabolism is fuelled almost exclusively by carbohydrate. Initially, this carbohydrate is derived from local stores of glycogen within the individual muscle cells. The total amount of glycogen available in the body is sufficient (in theory) for twelve hours at a sedentary metabolic rate. Alternatively, glycogen stores could support one hour of running at ten mph (six minute miles) — if all of it was available to the muscles carrying out this work. However, limited to using just its own internal glycogen resources, no muscle could support more than thirty minutes of moderate activity, and a much shorter duration of vigorous activity. Fig. 3.12 gives an example of work at 30% of maximum oxygen uptake (a very modest effort).

Other resources gradually become available to the working muscles. Within twenty minutes, half of their energy comes from glucose and fats carried in blood. Using glucose reduces its concentration in the blood and this reflexly reduces the production of insulin, the hormone which keeps blood sugar low after meals. Simultaneously another hormone, adrenaline, is secreted. The effects of these and other hormonal changes maintain normal blood glucose concentrations by stimulating the breakdown of glycogen in the liver. The glucose so formed is released into the bloodstream to replenish whatever the working muscles remove.

In addition to relying on stored glycogen to maintain blood

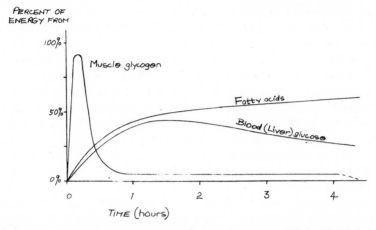

Fig. 3.12 In prolonged low intensity work, fats provide about half of the energy. As the work load increases, the proportion of energy supplied by fats decreases, reducing endurance. Near VO$_{2MAX}$ all of the energy for work is derived from carbohydrate and exhaustion is rapid.

glucose concentrations, the liver also takes lactic acid from the blood, and converts it into glucose, which is discharged back into the blood. Certain amino acids (protein fragments) can also be used to make glucose. Nevertheless, after an hour or so the liver's glycogen is partly depleted, and plasma concentrations of glucose begin to fall, reducing the amount available to muscle.

Only the body's fat stores have the resources to cater for long term endurance. Fat is made available or mobilised and released into the blood under the influence of noradrenaline, a potent stimulator of fat mobilisation. Noradrenaline appears in the blood both during brief intense exercise, and in moderate prolonged work. Fat is also mobilised by the same stimuli that release glucose from the liver — the increased adrenaline and decreased insulin concentrations which occur during exercise. Within an hour, the concentration of fats in the blood may have increased five-fold.

The use of fat for energy parallels that of liver-derived blood glucose during the first hour of moderate exercise (Fig. 3.12). Preference for fat is largely determined by its availability. As the glucose content of blood drops while that of fat rises, muscle turns increasingly to fat for energy. The consumption of sugary drinks or carbohydrate food prior to exercise raises blood glucose. This reflexly stimulates insulin secretion*, encouraging the use of glucose, delaying fat mobilisation, and hence (paradoxically) speeding glycogen depletion (see p. 190). There is also the danger of hypoglycaemic collapse. This comes about because BOTH exercise (by increasing adrenaline secretion) and insulin promote the removal of glucose from the blood, which can occur so rapidly that compensation is not possible. The low blood glucose concentration can then cause confusion and collapse.

Exhaustion occurs when glycogen reserves run short. (Of course, other factors may also terminate endurance exercise, such as circulatory failure — Ch. 6, or heat prostration — Ch. 7.) Blood glucose concentrations then begin to drop. The brain, which can only use glucose, ceases to function effectively as its fuel supply diminishes. In the example given (Fig. 3.12), with a modest work load of 30% of the person's maximum, this occurs after four hours. If the work load is increased, exhaustion of fuel reserves occurs earlier partly because less energy can be derived from fat (Fig. 3.13). Experienced marathon runners try to pace themselves so that exhaustion occurs as they cross the finish line. For well trained champions this will happen in just over two hours, while fun runners may have to endure over four hours!

Glycogen stores and the availability of glucose are important factors which place a limit on endurance. One key to developing endurance is to increase the glycogen stores. Another is to spare glucose by increased reliance on energy from fat instead.

Metabolic effects of endurance training

Endurance training occurs whenever a sufficiently strenuous activity is repeated for a sufficiently long time. In sedentary individuals relatively little effort is required to achieve an improvement. A minimum training effect can be seen if the activity elevates the heart rate to 130–140 beats per minute, for ten minutes, on three

---

* Diabetics either lack insulin, or fail to respond normally to the insulin they produce. During exercise, the rate of removal of glucose from the blood is greatly increased. For this reason, the dose of insulin (or other medication) a diabetic takes should be reduced on a day when exercise is contemplated. Diabetics should not undertake exercise without consulting their doctor.

PERCENT OF
FAT OXIDISED

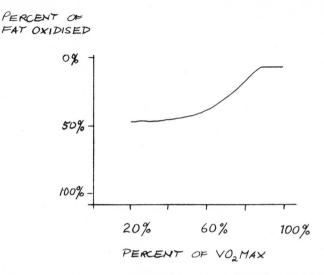

Fig. 3.13 *In prolonged work fat and carbohydrate share the provision of energy for work. The proportion of energy which comes from fat depends on the intensity of work.*

occasions per week. More obvious effects will be realised if the regime is harder, of longer duration, and more frequent. For the physically fit individual, vigorous training is required for any effect to be noted. Various training schedules have been proposed, with work intensities up to the VO_{2MAX} and with heart rates at 95% of maximum being recommended for athletes.

Ordinary mortals have to choose more modest regimes. One suggests that the heart rate during training should be maintained at the resting value plus 60% of the difference between the resting and the maximum value. This scheme gives oxygen consumptions of around 50% of VO_{2MAX} in untrained and 60% of VO_{2MAX} in trained people. For sedentary subjects starting a training programme, this is an energetic but realistic regime which should permit them to sustain the activity for about half an hour, long enough to give a good training effect.

There are two areas where training could have an effect on metabolism. One of these is in muscle where the ability to use fuel and oxygen might be improved, increasing the maximum work

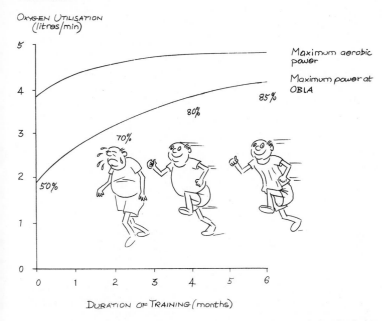

Oxygen Utilisation (litres/min)

Maximum aerobic power

Maximum power at OBLA

Fig. 3.14 Untrained individuals are able to sustain a work load of about half their VO$_{2MAX}$. As training proceeds, VO$_{2MAX}$ increases slightly, but the maximum sustainable work load increases dramatically and may reach 85% of VO$_{2MAX}$.

rate. The other possible improvement is in the ability of the body to mobilise and supply fuels and oxygen to the working muscles, increasing endurance.

effects of endurance training on VO$_{2MAX}$

Endurance training increases VO$_{2MAX}$ (Fig. 3.14). The increase achieved depends on the physical fitness of the individual before the start of training. Thus older, sedentary individuals can achieve spectacular gains of 30% in VO$_{2MAX}$ while younger, more active people might expect no more than a 10% improvement. On the other hand, lack of physical activity has the reverse effect, reducing VO$_{2MAX}$. Three weeks of bed rest has been shown to reduce VO$_{2MAX}$ by 25–30%.

Endurance training demands a high rate of metabolism. Some of the improvement in VO$_{2MAX}$ following training can be attributed to changes in the enzyme (biological catalysts) content of the cell. The enzymes involved in aerobic metabolism are located inside mitochondria, small membranous organs within cells. The total number of mitochondria increases, enhancing the ability of muscle to oxidise fuels. Since a similar increase in the numbers of mitochondria is seen in adaptation to high altitudes, their increase following training may be associated with the periodic lack of oxygen which a muscle must experience during strenuous work.

However, the reason why VO_{2MAX} responds to training is not properly understood. Much of the response may be simply due to the improved performance of the trained cardiovascular system (Ch. 6) which is better able to supply the working muscle. However, any increase in VO_{2MAX} probably plays only a small role in the greatly enhanced performance which follows training. Changes in other aspects of metabolism are far more important.

fat metabolism, the key to endurance
An evaluation of the body's energy resources (Fig. 3.4) quickly shows that, if endurance is to be developed, the use of fat as a fuel must be encouraged. Under normal circumstances, the body appears to be reluctant to use fat. Thus, fat makes little contribution to the energy requirements of brief bouts of activity. Moreover, as the intensity of activity increases, the proportion of energy supplied by fats diminishes (Fig. 3.13), and in strenuous work carbohydrate provides virtually all the energy.

Of course, the body is not really "reluctant" to use fat. Muscles remove approximately half of the fat the bloodstream brings them. At rest, the blood contains relatively little fat, limiting the use muscle can make of this fuel. During the early phase of an endurance activity, the availability of fat is poor leaving carbohydrate to provide most of the extra energy required. As activity continues, fat is mobilised from its depots, gradually taking over the supply of energy from carbohydrate. For the most part, this is due simply to the increasing availability to working muscle of fats in the blood.

Fat mobilisation is encouraged initially by a reduction in insulin and increase in noradrenaline secretion. Later, the secretion of growth hormone becomes important in maintaining fat availability. Although noradrenaline secretion begins with exercise, or even before, the mobilisation of fat takes time. One important change which follows endurance training is speeding up the process of fat mobilisation. Since their mobilisation of fat is faster, fat fuel is available sooner to trained individuals. They then use up less of their scarce glycogen reserves in the early phase of activity, and obtain a greater proportion of their energy from fat throughout exercise. This greatly increases endurance. The mechanisms behind faster fat mobilisation are not entirely understood, but the adipocytes (fat storage cells) may simply become more sensitive to noradrenaline, responding faster and more vigorously.

Fat mobilisation itself is not enough. There are various reasons why muscle tends to use carbohydrate instead of fat for energy in sedentary individuals. For a start, their muscle is relatively poorly equipped with the set of enzymes required to oxidise or burn fat. Training increases the quantity of fat metabolising enzymes in muscle, and hence its ability to use fat.

Producing ATP from fat instead of carbohydrate requires almost twice as much oxygen. At high rates of work muscle is always short of oxygen (Ch. 5) and this will bias it towards the use of glycogen rather than fat. Fat metabolism is relatively slow. Increasing the demand for ATP production will also favour the use of carbohydrate over fat. Furthermore, the presence of lactic acid, whose concentration rises at high work rates, inhibits fat metabolism.

Cardiovascular changes (Ch. 6) improve the delivery of oxygen to trained muscle. This makes available more oxygen and suppresses the production of lactic acid, both encouraging the use of fat. Finally, an improved supply of fat to muscle, brought by the increased rate of blood flow, will also stimulate its use.

In summary, a combination of:

1. faster and greater fat mobilisation from stores,
2. better blood flow in muscle, and
3. a higher concentration of the enzymes which catalyse fat metabolism all favour fat as a fuel over carbohydrate. The ability to burn fat at high rates uses an abundant fuel, conserving scarce carbohydrate and improving endurance. The increased metabolism of fat (always aerobic), plus an enhanced ability to metabolise carbohydrate aerobically reduces lactate production and accumulation. This also makes an important contribution to endurance and performance.

effects of endurance training on anaerobic threshold

Apart from success in suitable competition, probably the best index of the effectiveness of an endurance training programme is the anaerobic threshold. This is found by testing the subject at a series of graded workloads (on a treadmill or other ergometer) and measuring the concentration of lactic acid in blood after a short time at each load. The point at which this concentration reaches a predetermined value (usually 4 mmol/l — although other values are also used) is said to mark the Onset of Blood Lactate Accumulation, or OBLA (see p. 50).

Pyruvic acid (the precursor of lactic acid) is produced as the first stage of glucose metabolism, glycolysis. This step is anaerobic — requires no oxygen — and can proceed very rapidly if necessary. Normally, pyruvic acid feeds into the cell's aerobic metabolism, and doesn't accumulate. However, if the demand for energy (ATP) is particularly high, aerobic metabolism cannot cope, and the very fast anaerobic stage simply accelerates until demand is satisfied. The rate of production of pyruvic acid can exceed the ability of the muscle to metabolise it. Surplus pyruvic acid is converted into lactic acid which leaves the cell. The lactic acid concentration in the blood then begins to rise. When its concentration reaches 4 mmol/l, this is a sign that the other tissues which normally use it (mainly heart and kidney) can no longer cope with the amounts being produced. If the work load is increased further, the lactic acid concentration begins to rise steeply.

A high and rising concentration of lactic acid signals the approach of fatigue. A laboratory test can define the point of OBLA as a rate of oxygen consumption, a heart rate, or a level running speed for particular individuals. If they are asked to run in their own home neighbourhood with a heart rate monitor, it is clear that experienced athletes accurately and instinctively sense the work load which corresponds to their own anaerobic threshold, and pace themselves accordingly, so that their heart rates are reasonably steady. When novice runners are similarly tested, their heart rates are far more erratic.

Untrained individuals are able to work at a load corresponding to approximately half of their VO_{2MAX} before the lactic acid concentration in their blood reaches 4 mmol/l. After several months of endurance training, the same subjects could expect to achieve work loads of 75–80% of VO_{2MAX} before lactic acid begins to accumulate in the body. The graph (Fig. 3.14) shows that several months of training produces a very substantial improvement in anaerobic threshold, although the parallel increase in VO_{2MAX} is modest.

what does anaerobic threshold mean to me?

The improvement in OBLA with training translates into the ability to maintain a higher rate of energy expenditure than before without encountering fatigue. Prior to training, the same rate of energy expenditure would have required anaerobic metabolism, which would have generated lactic acid. The onset of fatigue is hastened by lactic acid accumulation. Producing ATP aerobically avoids this contribution to fatigue, improving endurance.

Fatigue is also caused by the depletion of muscle and liver glygogen. By relying more heavily on fat metabolism for the production of ATP, glycogen stores are conserved, increasing endurance. Probably even more important is the effect of minimising anaerobic metabolism. Aerobically metabolised, a unit of glycogen can generate nearly twenty times as much ATP as it could anaerobically. The lactic acid produced then leaves the muscle. When lactic acid leaves, its energy is not lost from the body, but it represents a substantial loss of energy reserves from that muscle, reducing its endurance.

Summary

Endurance training increases the maximum rate at which ATP can be generated. Also improved is the rate at which ATP can be generated on a continuous basis. This increase occurs only in the muscles which have been affected by the training regime.

Probably even more important are changes in the metabolic processes involved in ATP production. There is greater reliance on aerobic metabolism and on the use of fat as a fuel instead of carbohydrate. This conserves glycogen stores and increases endurance. Reliance on aerobic processes reduces the export of lactic acid from the working muscles and conserves their glycogen stores, enhancing endurance.

Normally, aerobic metabolism is limited by the ability of the cardiovascular system to deliver oxygen. This is particularly so if fat is being used as a fuel since ATP production demands more oxygen to burn fat than carbohydrate. So the above changes must proceed hand in hand with improvements in the ability of the cardiovascular system to deliver oxygen (Ch. 6).

CHAPTER FOUR

Respiratory physiology

The purpose of the respiratory system is to bring the blood into intimate contact with atmospheric air so that oxygen can be absorbed and carbon dioxide given up. Every day, the respiratory system extracts about 360 litres of oxygen from some 10,000 litres of air. Working as hard as it can, the respiratory system of a 70 kg man can remove four litres of oxygen from 150 litres of air each minute. It is particularly important that the respiratory system accomplishes this without exposing the moist, delicate tissues where gas exchange occurs to either physical damage or to drying.

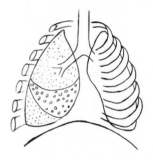

The respiratory system consists of a pair of lungs, connected to the atmosphere via the bronchi and trachea, the whole enclosed within the ribs and muscles of the chest (Fig. 4.1), and controlled by a respiratory centre in the brain. Unlike the heart, which beats spontaneously, the respiration ceases in the absence of commands from the brain.

Fig. 4.1 The lungs are enclosed within a cage formed by the ribs and the respiratory muscles, and connected to the atmosphere via the trachea and bronchi.

Anatomy of the respiratory system

The trachea (windpipe) is a semi-rigid tube leading from the larynx in the middle of the neck to the point where it divides into the two bronchi, one leading to each lung. The trachea and bronchi are composed of sections of cartilage shaped like a letter "C" (these can be felt low in the neck) (Fig. 4.2a). These are bound

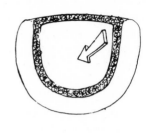

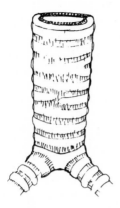

Fig. 4.2a The trachea and bronchi are reinforced by rings of cartilage.

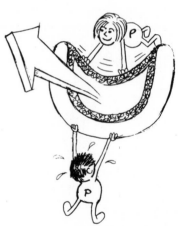

Fig. 4.2b The cartilage rings are "C" shaped. While preventing collapse under moderate pressure, the unreinforced side can bulge inwards under the high pressure (P) of a cough, greatly increasing velocity so that obstructions may be blown away.

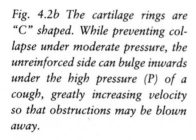

together with muscle and connective tissue, and lined with mucosal tissue. The cartilage is flexible, but serves to keep the bronchi from collapsing under any pressure changes (Fig. 4.2b) to which they may be subjected. The muscle can contract, constricting the smaller bronchi and reducing their cross-section. Such constriction, induced by irritants or allergens, is responsible for asthma. In coughing, high pressure is developed in the chest. This invaginates the large airways (see diagram) so that a particularly high velocity of air flow may be achieved, which can then blow away any accumulated mucus and debris.

The two main bronchi subdivide 23 times, eventually yielding eight million terminal bronchioles in each lung, each less than 1 mm in diameter. Although individual bronchioles are small, there are many of them, and the total cross-section area is very large, much larger than in the trachea. The velocity of flow is highest in the trachea, and decreases in the smaller bronchioles where the cross-section area is greatest (see below).

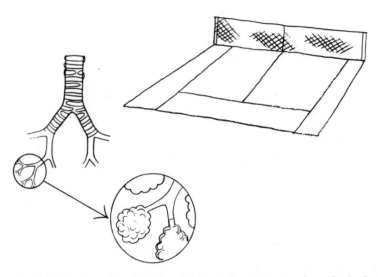

Fig. 4.3 The bronchi subdivide, ultimately becoming tiny bronchioles less than 1 mm in diameter. These terminate in grape-like clusters of tiny sacs called alveoli. The total surface area of alveoli in both lungs is as large as half a tennis court.

The terminal bronchioles each give rise to 30–40 thin-walled sacs called alveoli which cluster around the bronchioles like bunches of grapes. There is a total of 600 million alveoli in both lungs. This is where gas (carbon dioxide and oxygen) exchange occurs. Although the total gas volume of both lungs is only six litres, the surface area of the alveoli is estimated to be 70–100 m^2, or half the area of a singles tennis court, a remarkable feat of packaging.

Each alveolus is about 0.3 mm diameter and made up of a single layer of thin epithelial cells with some connective tissue binding them together. Each alveolus has a dense network of

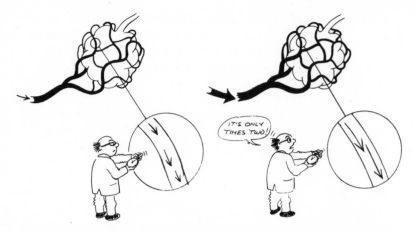

Fig. 4.4 The surface of an alveolus is covered with blood capillaries. During exercise, lung blood flow increases five-fold but, because more capillaries come into use, the velocity of flow only doubles.

capillaries embedded within itself, bringing deoxygenated venous blood from the body for oxygenation. About half the surface area of the alveolus is covered with capillaries (Fig. 4.4)

This soft tissue is packed into the chest, surrounding the heart. The chest itself is made of the bony ribs, which are bound together by the intercostal muscles. The top of the chest is closed off by the collarbone and its associated muscles. The bottom of the chest is sealed by a muscular sheet called the diaphragm. The chest is lined with a smooth, slippery pleural membrane, and the surface of the lung is also wrapped in this membrane. These membranes are in close contact, separated by the fluid-filled pleural space.

Mechanics of respiration

The chest cavity can be increased and decreased in volume, and breathing is accomplished by these volume changes. Volume is increased when the diaphragm contracts and flattens, increasing the height of the chest (Fig. 4.5). Contraction of the external intercostal muscles lifts the ribs (Fig. 4.6a), increasing the diameter of the chest. Together these changes enlarge the volume of the chest. When the volume of the chest increases, the pressure in the

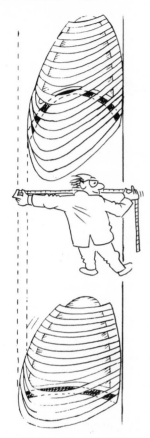

Fig. 4.5 During inspiration the ribs rise, increasing the diameter of the chest. At the same time the diaphragm (dark shading) contracts, flattening and increasing the height of the chest cavity. These two actions lower pressure within the chest, causing air to enter the lungs via the bronchi.

pleural space decreases. The alveoli and terminal bronchioles are elastic. They are readily stretched by this negative pressure, drawing air in.

The reverse manoeuvre, allowing the diaphragm to relax and contracting the internal intercostal muscles, diminishes the volume of the chest. However, in normal quiet breathing, the expiratory muscles are not actually used. Instead, as the inspiratory muscles relax, the elastic recoil of the chest and alveoli causes the lungs to deflate (Fig. 4.6b). When breathing becomes more vigorous, the expiratory muscles are brought into play, increasing the pressure within the pleural space and speeding lung deflation.

lung protection
When air is drawn in, dust and other foreign matter accompanies it. Because the velocity of flow decreases markedly as the air travels down to the smallest bronchioles, any inhaled dust particles tend to settle. These are caught on the mucus coating the respiratory passages well before reaching the alveoli. The respiratory passages are lined with cells which are equipped with cilia, which are movable hair-like projections. These beat continuously at about 15 times per second. Their beating action sweeps mucus upwards at 1 cm/min towards the top of the trachea, from where it can be

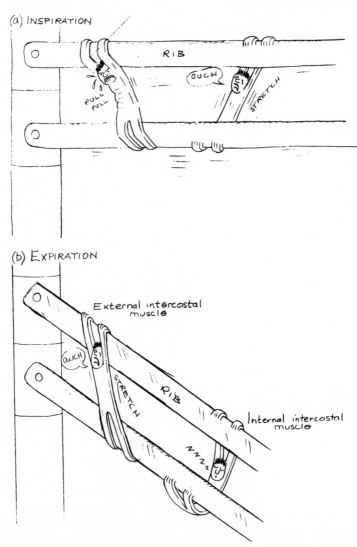

Fig. 4.6 (a) The ribs are hinged at the spine. The external intercostal muscles are so arranged that their contraction lifts the ribs. Meanwhile the internal intercostal muscles are stretched, providing one of the signals which stops inspiration (see Fig. 4.14).
(b) In quiet breathing the ribs simply fall as the external intercostal muscles relax. During exercise, contraction of the internal intercostal muscles forces the ribs down, vigorously emptying the lungs.

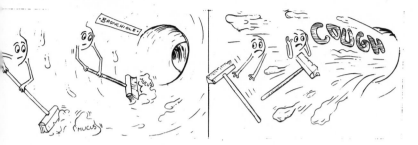

Fig. 4.7 *The respiratory passages are lined with ciliated cells. The cilia move rhythmically, sweeping mucus (constantly secreted locally) upwards towards the trachea. If mucus and any debris caught in it accumulate, a cough blows this obstruction upwards to the oesophagus where it can be swallowed or spat out.*

coughed up if it accumulates. Small amounts of mucus are swallowed unconsciously throughout the day. Around 10–100 ml of mucus are produced every day, depending on irritation, infection, etc.

Before atmospheric air can be allowed to reach the alveoli, it must be moistened to 100% humidity or the moist alveolar tissue would rapidly dry and die. This humidification is carried out by evaporating water from the nose, mouth, and upper respiratory passages. In cold climates, a combination of the very cold air and evaporation of water can make breathing quite painful.

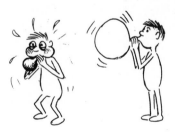

Fig. 4.8

surface tension

Party balloons are initially difficult to inflate, but after the first puff of air enters and they enlarge, further inflation becomes far easier. This is explained by the Law of Laplace (Fig. 4.9).

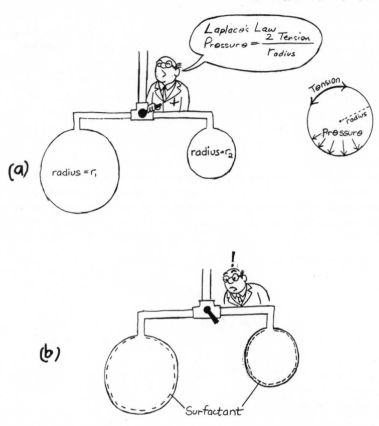

Fig. 4.9 (a) The Law of Laplace states that if two balloons with identical properties have different sizes, the one with the smaller radius must have a greater pressure inside. If they are connected together via the valve, the smaller will collapse into the larger.

(b) However, if the balloons are bubbles coated with surfactant (as the alveoli are), this reduces surface tension. Moreover, as the balloon shrinks, the surfactant coating it becomes more concentrated, further dropping surface tension. If the two balloons are now connected, neither collapses. The presence of surfactant allows alveoli of various sizes to co-exist without collapsing.

The smaller the radius of the balloon, the greater the pressure required to prevent its collapse — despite the fact that a smaller radius means less stretch and less elastic tension in the rubber wall. Alveoli are not rubber and their epithelial cells are not elastic. However, they are wet and watery bubbles and develop a surface tension which tries to collapse them. (Surface tension causes water to form round droplets on a waxed or greasy surface.) Surface tension provides most of the elastic recoil of lung tissue. Alveoli secrete a detergent-like substance (surfactant or surface active agent). Detergents reduce surface tension, making possible the long term survival of bubbles in the bath.

In the lung the tendency of alveoli to collapse is almost eliminated by the surfactant. If the alveoli collapsed, they would have to be reinflated at every breath, at great effort. Fortunately, most people have to make this effort just once, at birth. Surfactant also stabilises the lung, allowing alveoli of different sizes to co-exist. Lack of surfactant in the lungs of premature infants increases the work of breathing and can give rise to the sometimes fatal Respiratory Distress Syndrome.

work in breathing

Apart from alveolar surface tension, a second elastic force is provided by the chest wall, which has a preferred volume and shape. Any enlargement or decrease in size requires work to be done against these elastic forces.

Work must also be done to overcome the friction of air movement through the respiratory passages. This increases very steeply with the velocity of flow. The velocity increases in exercise, but particularly in diseases where the airways are constricted such as asthma. Atmospheric pollution may irritate the airways, causing them to constrict and increasing the work of breathing. Ozone is usually the chief pollutant involved (see p. 76 for effects on athletic performance).

The work of breathing is the sum of the work done against the elastic forces of the chest and lung, and that done against the friction of air movement in the respiratory passages. In quiet breathing, energy is expended only during inspiration. At rest, expiration is passive and accomplished by the release of elastic tension. During exercise, the work of breathing may rise 20-fold, and some of this work must be done by the expiratory muscles.

Lung volumes

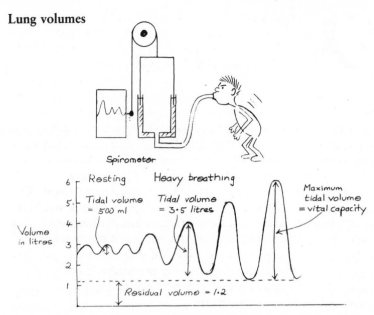

Fig. 4.10 (a) The spirometer bell floats on water as pictured. Breathing into the device makes it move, recording the volumes breathed on a paper-covered drum.
(b) In normal quiet breathing the volume moved (the tidal volume) is around 500 ml. As respiratory movements become more vigorous, the volume moved increases.

In quiet breathing, about 500 ml of air moves at each breath. This is the "tidal volume". As oxygen consumption goes up, the tidal volume rises. At first just the volume of air inspired increases. In hard work when expiration becomes active the expiratory volume also increases contributing to the expansion in tidal volume (Fig. 4.10). Following a maximum inspiration with complete expiration gives the "vital capacity", a measure of the usable lung volume. This is typically 4.5 litres in a 70 kg man and 3 litres in a 60 kg woman. The vital capacity decreases with age (probably due to greater stiffness of the chest), and between the ages of 20 and 60 a man can expect a 20% loss, while a woman will lose 15%. Diseases such as pneumonia can permanently reduce vital capacity. However, unless more than 25% of the lung volume is lost, the patient is unlikely to be aware of any problem.

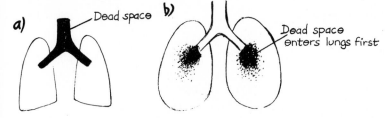

Fig. 4.11 *The respiratory passages are filled with gas from the last expiration. This volume is called the dead space and is first to enter the lungs on the next inspiration.*

At the beginning of each inspiration, the airways are filled with "stale" air — the end of the preceding expiration. This is called the dead space and is equal to the volume of the airways (Fig. 4.11). The dead space volume ranges from 100–200 ml and reduces the useful tidal volume. As a rough guide, the dead space in millilitres is equal to the body weight in pounds. Thus, with a breath of 500 ml, the actual volume of fresh air entering the lungs of a 70 kg (159 lbs) person is about 350 ml. As breathing becomes deeper, the dead space remains the same, and the efficiency of respiration improves slightly.

Even after a forced expiration, about one litre of air remains in the lungs. This is termed the residual volume and its existence saves a great deal of respiratory work. Its absence would imply collapse of the alveoli at each expiration and the need to re-inflate them from zero volume, like party balloons. The existence of both the dead space and the residual volume also reduces the changes in blood gas concentration during breathing (see below). Residual volume increases with age, starting at 20% of vital capacity at age 20 and rising to 30% by age 60.

The amount of air which is breathed each minute is termed the Minute Volume. However, some of this is used to ventilate the dead space. The amount of air passing through the alveoli each minute is termed Alveolar Ventilation:

ALVEOLAR VENTILATION = (MINUTE VOLUME)
    − (DEAD SPACE VENTILATION)

respiratory "efficiency"
Inefficiency in breathing is partly due to the dead space, but

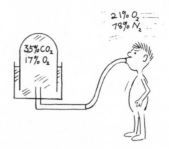

Fig. 4.12 In quiet breathing, the composition of the expired air is approximately 17% oxygen and 3.5% carbon dioxide.

mainly to the small fraction of the lung volume which is ventilated at each breath. The transfer of oxygen from lungs to blood depends on maintaining a high concentration of the gas in the alveoli. If this were to drop, it would not be possible to load blood fully with oxygen (Ch. 5). This requirement strictly limits the amount of oxygen which can be extracted from the air breathed, and hence the respiratory efficiency. It is possible to estimate the ventilation required to support various work loads.

Atmospheric air is 21% oxygen, 78% nitrogen, with traces of carbon dioxide and other gases. In the alveoli, the oxygen is partly removed, while carbon dioxide and water vapour are added. At rest, the expired gas consists of 17% oxygen and 3.5% carbon dioxide (Fig. 4.12). The amount of oxygen removed is:

$$21\% - 17\% = 4\%,$$

and,

$$(21\% - 17\%)/21\% \times 100 = 19\%,$$

or 19% of the oxygen in the air is extracted.

Since air contains 21% oxygen, the volume of oxygen removed from the air (or the breathing efficiency) is:

$$0.21 \times 0.19 \times 100 = 4\%.$$

This means that only 4% of the volume of air breathed actually goes to support metabolism.

The normal resting oxygen consumption is 250 ml/min. In order to obtain this amount of oxygen (with an efficiency of 4%), a person must breathe:

250/0.04 = 6250 ml/min = 6.3 litres of air per minute.

As oxygen consumption increases and breathing becomes deeper, efficiency improves slightly, but it never rises much, and during exercise the expired air still contains 15.5% oxygen, giving an oxygen extraction of:

$$(21\% - 15.5\%)/21\% \times 100 = 26\%,$$

and a breathing efficiency of:

$$0.26 \times 0.21 \times 100 = 5.5\%.$$

So, to support an oxygen consumption of two litres per min,

$$2/0.055 = 36 \text{ litres per minute}$$

of air should be breathed. For reasons which will be explained elsewhere efficiency falls again at high work loads, and respiratory minute volumes (volume of air breathed per minute) of over 150 litres per minute may be needed to support the maximum oxygen consumption of a normal 70 kg man (about four litres per minute).

respiratory performance

At a resting oxygen consumption of 250 ml per minute, the respiratory minute volume will be about six litres per minute. If the respiratory rate is twelve breaths per minute, the tidal volume will be 500 ml. Both the respiratory rate and the tidal volume increase substantially to support high metabolic rates.

Although the vital capacity may be five litres, the extremes of volume at maximum inspiration and expiration cannot be used because of the time and effort it takes to achieve them. If you try to completely fill, and then totally empty your lungs, you will quickly appreciate this. In practice, the maximum useful tidal volume is around 3.5 litres. Higher volumes fail to increase the minute volume due to reduction in respiratory rate.

The respiratory rate has no clear maximum. The faster the respiration rate, the greater the work done against the forces of inertia to accelerate the ribs, muscles, diaphragm, etc. as they alternate between inspiration and expiration.* A limit is reached

---

* Some animals (sheep, dogs) pant at specific rates which may exceed 200 per minute. Such high rates are only possible because their respiratory machinery resonates at the panting frequency. In panting, the tidal volume becomes very small so that little air is moved and the composition of the blood gases is not disturbed.

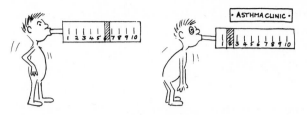

Fig. 4.13 One simple measure of respiratory performance is the Peak Expiratory Flow Rate (PEFR). This is the highest rate of expiratory flow which can be achieved by the person being tested.

at 40–60 breaths per minute. Higher rates are costly in terms of work, and actually fail to increase minute volume due to diminishing tidal volume.

Another important measure of respiratory performance is the resistance of the airways (trachea, bronchi, etc.) to flow. At rest, the flow resistance is very low. This is commonly measured by doctors as the peak expiratory flow rate (PEFR) using a cheap and simple hand-held device into which the subject blows as hard as possible (Fig. 4.13). A typical value is 600 litres per minute for a man and 450 litres per minute for a woman. This is a very high rate of air flow and is obviously attained only very briefly. In a hospital, measurements might be made of the speed at which air can be exhaled, or the Forced Expiratory Volume in one second (FEV1). The subject takes a maximum breath and exhales as fast as possible. It is normally possible to exhale at least 80% of the vital capacity in one second. Both the PEFR and the FEV1 deteriorate with age as the tissues making up the respiratory system lose their elasticity.

Disease can greatly reduce respiratory performance, but it is remarkable by how much it must deteriorate before the patient becomes aware of the problem. Thus asthmatics commonly reach values of PEFR as low as 150–200 litres per minute before complaining of wheezing. Clearly, active individuals tend to be more sensitive to wheezing than sedentary people.

Certain atmospheric pollutants, of which ozone is the most important, irritate the airways and reduce the PEFR (the effect is far greater in asthmatics and other sensitive people). Respiratory performance does not normally affect athletic performance. However, a study of the outcome of competitive long distance races in

Californian secondary school students over a five year period produced an interesting result. There was a good correlation between atmospheric ozone in the hour before the race and running performance. There was a poorer correlation with suspended particles, and none with carbon monoxide.

matching lung blood flow with ventilation

The two lungs receive the same total blood flow as the rest of the body. However, the resistance to flow of the lung blood vessels is lower than that of the rest of the body and the pulmonary arterial blood pressure is low, which is why the right ventricle is less muscular than the left (Ch. 6).

Oxygen depleted blood enters the lung, and on passing through an alveolus, becomes oxygenated. However, if blood should pass through a poorly ventilated alveolus (whose bronchiole is blocked with mucus), this oxygen-depleted blood would then mix with oxygenated blood and decrease the oxygen content of arterial blood. This is ventilation–perfusion mismatching.

Fortunately, poor ventilation and its sequel, low oxygen content, usually causes nearby alveolar blood vessels to constrict, reducing their blood flow. This response diverts blood away from the blocked alveoli and minimises the amount of deoxygenated blood which is able to enter the arterial supply. The reverse problem is ventilation of an alveolus which receives little blood flow. Unless it is extensive, the latter type of mismatching has little physiological consequence.

Blood flow tends to be low at the top of the lung where the pulmonary arterial pressure is least (due to gravity) and high at the base of the lung where the pressure is greater. At rest the tidal volume is so small that many alveoli are poorly ventilated. Most of these poorly ventilated alveoli are located at the top of the lung (where the chest is stiffer), which tends to match ventilation and blood flow quite well. Consequently, the blood leaving the lungs of normal individuals at rest usually carries 95% of its maximum oxygen capacity.

As soon as exercise begins, the increased vigour of respiration tends to bring poorly ventilated alveoli into use. Simultaneously, the increase in cardiac output raises the pulmonary arterial blood pressure. This improves the flow to the top of the lung where low pressure normally restricts flow at rest. The matching of ventilation and flow improves in exercise so that blood leaving the lungs now carries 98–100% of its oxygen-carrying capacity.

Control of respiration

chemical control — carbon dioxide
The main waste product of metabolic activity is carbon dioxide which, when dissolved in water, becomes carbonic acid. The accumulation of acid in the bloodstream would rapidly upset the body's normal pH (a logarithmic measure of the amount of acid in solution: pH = 7.0 is neutral, and the mildly alkaline pH = 7.4 is normal for arterial blood), and stop metabolism, which would cause death. The body has two routes for the excretion of acid — the kidney and the lungs. Each day, the respiratory system gets rid of 200 times as much acid as do the kidneys, and could dispose of much more if necessary.

Since the amount of dissolved carbon dioxide is a major factor determining the pH of the blood, rapid control of pH is achieved by adjusting its loss through breathing. The body has devices which measure both pH and carbon dioxide concentration. These

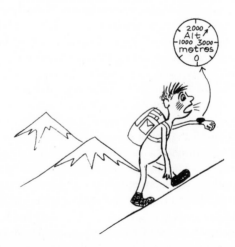

Fig. 4.14 *At high altitudes atmospheric pressure falls, and oxygen partial pressure falls with it. At 2500 metres above sea level, the oxygen partial pressure is low enough to stimulate respiration at rest, and to hinder performance in activity.*

are called chemoreceptors and are located in the brain's blood supply (some in the neck, others in the brain itself).

If the metabolic rate rises, more carbon dioxide is produced and its concentration in blood begins to rise. The chemoreceptors detect this change and stimulate breathing. Increasing lung ventilation speeds the loss or "blows off" more carbon dioxide, restoring normal pH.

chemical control — oxygen

Oxygen also has a role in respiratory control. There are chemoreceptors in the carotid arteries leading to the brain which measure the oxygen content of the arterial blood. When the oxygen content of blood falls, they stimulate respiration increasing ventilation to bring more oxygen into the lungs. Chemoreceptors are however, relatively insensitive to changes in the partial pressure* of atmospheric oxygen. This is partly due to the oxygen-carrying characteristics of haemoglobin (Ch. 5), and partly to the way in which the receptors work.

The oxygen chemoreceptors become stimulated in an oxygen-poor environment (eg: a submarine which has been submerged for several hours). Stimulation also occurs at high altitudes due to the drop in atmospheric pressure which reduces the partial pressure of oxygen. The first sign of such stimulation is normally seen at around 8000 feet altitude (2500 m). Here atmospheric pressure is 25% lower than at sea level. The partial pressure of oxygen in the lung and the blood decreases, mildly stimulating respiration. Despite this, the oxygen content of arterial blood is reduced by about 10%.

At 10,000 ft altitude and higher, problems begin to occur. The rate of ventilation which is adequate to vent the carbon dioxide generated at rest is too low to oxygenate blood normally in the thin air. The oxygen chemoreceptor stimulates breathing to bring more oxygen into the lung. This blows off too much carbon dioxide and upsets the blood pH. The carbon dioxide chemoreceptor stops breathing to correct pH, and then the oxygen receptor stimulates breathing to improve oxygenation ... This

---

* Since oxygen is 21% of atmospheric air, its partial pressure will be 21% of atmospheric pressure. So if the atmospheric pressure at sea level is 1000 millibars (mb), oxygen partial pressure will be 210 mb. On a mountainside, the atmospheric pressure might be 600 mb, and the oxygen partial pressure would then be 126 mb.

stop–go pattern of respiration is called Cheyne–Stokes breathing, and is characteristic of a first (generally sleepless) night spent at high altitude. In 15–20 hours, the loss from the blood, and the fluid bathing the brain, of some sodium bicarbonate (an alkali) allows the blood carbon dioxide (an acid) to stay low (due to the extra breathing) while the pH remains normal. Following this adjustment, a high rate of ventilation can be maintained to improve oxygenation. Just as a ship cannot have two captains, the abdication of responsibility by the oxygen chemoreceptor at or near sea level aids good control of breathing.

mechanical control
There are also mechanical controls of respiration. The respiratory muscles have built-in length measuring devices called stretch receptors (these are present in all skeletal muscles). The alveoli also have stretch receptors. During inspiration, the inspiratory muscles contract, and the expiratory muscles and alveoli are passively stretched (Fig. 4.15). This stretch is signalled to the brain, which stops inspiration and initiates expiration when an appropriate level of inflation is reached. This is the Hering–Breuer reflex, which automatically adjusts the depth of breathing as appropriate to the body's requirement for ventilation. At a resting minute volume of six litres per minute the tidal volume is set near 500 ml.

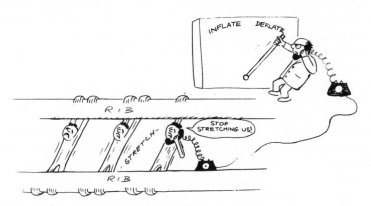

Fig. 4.15 During inspiration the ribs rise and the expiratory muscles become stretched. This passive stretch is signalled to the brain which stops inspiration at the appropriate point. Stretch signals from the alveoli are also monitored.

When the required minute volume is thirty litres per minute, the tidal volume is set at around 1.5 litres.

Mechanical control of respiration is also determined by the type of activity. This is discussed below (p. 85).

In summary, the control of respiration is mainly geared to maintain a constant carbon dioxide and pH in arterial blood. However, other information is also used and integrated in our normal fully automatic system. We can also take over conscious control for short periods of time.

Respiration in exercise

During exercise, the metabolic rate can rise by sixteen-fold above the resting value. This means that sixteen times as much oxygen must be taken up by the lungs, and sixteen times as much carbon dioxide must be excreted from the body.

Both processes are vital. Although some tissues in the body (such as muscles, intestine, & skin) are capable of anaerobic metabolism and can do without oxygen for quite long periods of time, the brain cannot survive more than five minutes in its absence and consciousness is lost in two to three minutes. So the supply of oxygen must remain adequate and continuous.

Carbon dioxide also cannot be allowed to accumulate in the body. Carbon dioxide dissolves readily in the blood and in other body fluids, forming carbonic acid. Although the blood can buffer the accumulation of acid, even the best buffers cannot entirely prevent the pH from changing. Again, the brain, which is particularly fussy about the acidity of its blood supply, is the weak link. Even a small change in the pH of the blood, either up or down, can cause unconsciousness.

Accordingly, respiratory activity must be closely and continuously matched to the body's activity. Excessive breathing or hyperventilation is as damaging as too little. The rate and depth of breathing is constantly adjusted as activity and the metabolic rate change.

respiratory performance in exercise
At rest, approximately six litres of air per minute are moved through the lungs. This is accomplished with breaths of about a half litre, some twelve times per minute, although this can vary

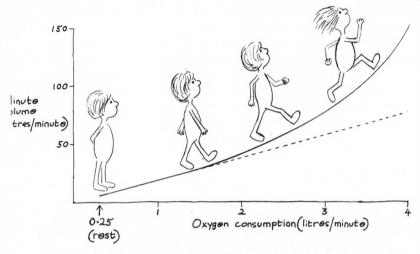

Fig. 4.16 *As work load increases and oxygen consumption rises, respiration is stimulated. The stimulation is proportional to oxygen consumption until the work load becomes high enough for lactic acid to accumulate in the blood (see Ch. 3).*

widely between individuals. During exercise, ventilation can increase to well over 100 litres per minute, with breaths of over three litres, 30–40 times per minute (Fig. 4.16). In contrast to the cardiovascular system's relatively modest five-fold increase in performance, the respiratory system is capable of a 25-fold increase. In well trained athletes at work lung ventilation can top 200 litres per minute, representing an increase of more than thirty times.

It is clear that lung ventilation is linearly related to metabolic rate and oxygen utilisation at low levels of activity. As the metabolic rate continues to increase, ventilation rises by more than would be expected. This response is due to the increasing contribution of anaerobic processes to the metabolic rate. Anaerobic metabolism produces lactic acid (Ch. 3). To compensate for the accumulation of this acid, respiration accelerates to blow off more carbon dioxide. This maintains body pH by reducing carbonic acid in the blood.

Breathing requires work. At rest, the respiratory muscles cost the body very little to operate. In order to supply one litre of oxygen to the body they consume a mere 0.5 ml of oxygen, or about 0.2% of the resting metabolic rate. By contrast, the work of the heart costs the body about seven per cent of the resting metabolic rate. In very hard work breathing costs 10% of the resting metabolic rate, while the heart uses 25%. So, compared to rest, in hard work the cost of breathing increases by fifty-fold while the cost of pumping blood rises just 3.5 times. However, the energy cost of breathing is low compared to that of pumping blood around the body.

is respiration limiting in exercise?

The rapid increase in the metabolic cost of respiration during exercise has prompted the question of whether the respiratory system could limit athletic performance. Normally the answer to this is no.

As activity increases, ventilation rises to match the body's requirement for oxygen and for carbon dioxide removal. The relationship between oxygen consumption and lung ventilation has the shape of a hockey stick. As the work load increases and oxygen consumption approaches maximum for that individual (VO_{2max}), ventilation begins to soar. At VO_{2max}, it is still possible for a physically fit individual to further increase work output, and with no change in oxygen consumption (which is already maximal). However, there is a further, often substantial, increase in ventilation. This strongly suggests that oxygen consumption is limited by some factor other than ventilation. (Additional work output beyond the point of VO_{2max} is met by anaerobic metabolism, — see Ch. 3. This level of work cannot be sustained for more than a few minutes.)

Another experiment indicates that the respiratory system is not limiting in exercise. A group of well trained athletes were asked to work at near their VO_{2max} for ten minutes. Part-way through the test, they were asked to deliberately hyperventilate and produced increases in ventilation averaging 13%. Moreover, in a separate test maximum ventilation was measured and found to be 33% greater than the ventilation at VO_{2max}. These results suggest that ventilation could not have been limiting performance.

Muscles become fatigued. Does fatigue of the respiratory muscles ever become a problem for endurance athletes? It has been demonstrated that, after an endurance race, athletes' performance in PEFR and FEV1 tests was poorer than it had been before the

D

start. This suggests that respiratory muscles can become fatigued, but there is no evidence that this fatigue actually limits track performance. Respiratory muscle fatigue is often experienced by unacclimatised individuals walking at high altitude. While the leg muscles probably work less hard than usual, the respiratory muscles must move far more air through the lungs to extract the required oxygen from the "thin" air. Although performance may be poor due to reduced oxygen availability, there is no evidence that respiratory muscle fatigue has contributed to this. On the other hand, certain atmospheric pollutants may affect performance by increasing the work of breathing (see p. 76).

Another potential limitation is in the rate at which oxygen and carbon dioxide diffuse across the lung to enter the blood. At rest, the blood entering an alveolus becomes fully saturated (loaded) with oxygen by the time it has completed one third of its journey through the capillary. In exercise, the heart's output increases five-fold. However, because more capillaries open providing parallel channels for flow, the velocity of flow barely doubles. This enables blood to become fully oxygenated by the time it has completed two thirds of its journey through an alveolar capillary. Carbon dioxide diffuses much more rapidly than oxygen and its transport is complete within 10–20% of the length of an alveolar capillary.

A likely reason why the respiratory system is designed with more capacity than appears to be required may be related to the frequency with which humans catch respiratory ailments. Perhaps the system is built to cope with these periods of subnormal performance without endangering survival.

Effects of training

Working a system usually improves it. In Peru, people have been living at altitudes of over 15,000 ft for thousands of years, herding livestock and mining silver. Since the air pressure at that altitude is reduced to about 60% of its sea level value, the lung ventilation required to satisfy one's need for oxygen is increased by more than 30%. Natives of the Peruvian Andes, therefore, all have well trained respiratory systems. It is not surprising that they have lung volumes which are 30–35% larger than genetically similar sea level natives.

However, examination of the respiratory performance of male

endurance athletes reveals small, but not statistically significant, differences compared to sedentary men of similar size and age:

	Runners	Sedentary
Vital capacity (litres)	5.9	5.1
FEV1 (litres)	4.8	4.2
FEV1/VC (%)	82	81
Residual volume (litres)	2.2	1.9

Similarly, Peruvian lowlanders who migrated to the uplands to work in Peru's high altitude silver mines have shown little change in respiratory performance, even after years in their new homes. This suggests that training does not enlarge the adult respiratory system, and may not even enhance performance. It is possible that the chest cavity may be incapable of further change after puberty when the bones cease to grow. (The chest does appear to enlarge in emphysema, a serious disease associated with smoking.)

Moreover, the performance of the respiratory system may make little or no difference to the work capacity of the individual. The respiratory system does not appear to be taxed to capacity during even the heaviest exercise.

Control of respiration in exercise

The mechanisms controlling respiration during exercise are poorly understood. It is widely believed that respiration is regulated with a view to maintaining a constant blood pH and carbon dioxide concentration. However, the system does this so well that these two parameters remain almost unchanged from rest to moderately hard work — so what can the body measure to acquire the information enabling it to control respiration with such great precision?

Every muscle, joint, and tendon constantly sends data in the form of nerve signals to the brain. This tells the brain precisely where each limb is in relation to the head and the other limbs, enabling us to perform many complex tasks without visual control. Thus, apart from bumping into unseen objects, we have no difficulty walking in total darkness.

Increase in the actvity of the limbs is known to stimulate respiration, and may also play an important role in its control. Thus, a pattern of activity such as walking up stairs or sawing

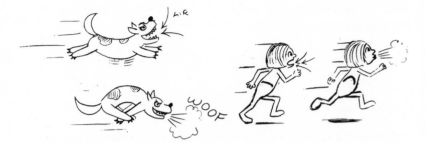

Fig. 4.17 Respiratory movements are often synchronised to body movements. In a running dog flexing of the body, while in a running human, gravity causes the diaphragm to drop, both of which assist respiration.

wood may rapidly call up a memorised ventilation rate, which has proved to supply enough oxygen in the past. Should the chemoreceptors monitoring blood oxygen and carbon dioxide report that activity and respiration are inadequately matched on a particular occasion, adjustments in ventilation may be made to correct this. The new respiratory response could then be used to update the remembered settings.

Another mechanical control of respiration is determined by the activity. Birds have no choice but to breathe in time with their wing beats because their flight muscles are wrapped around their chest, squeezing it with every contraction. Running dogs lengthen their stride by alternately curving and straightening their spine, again imposing a rhythm on their respiratory movements.

In running humans, every footfall causes the diaphragm and abdominal contents to drop, part of an inspiratory effort which runners make use of by synchronising inspiration to a footfall. The typical pattern is 2–3 paces per breath in level running, and less running uphill. This synchronisation saves effort. Activities like bicycling impose little mechanical constraint on respiration, while swimming imposes different ones.

Summary

During exercise, the metabolic rate can increase sixteen-fold and lung ventilation must increase by at least that much to supply the oxygen required and to remove the carbon dioxide produced. In fact, respiration increases far more than sixteen times, because additional carbon dioxide is lost to compensate for lactic acid accumulation during hard work. Physical training appears to do little or nothing to improve respiratory performance, nor is any improvement required since the system is usually only moderately stressed during even the hardest work. Control of respiration during exercise may be accomplished by registering the activity of the limbs, assigning an approximate ventilation rate from memory, and adjusting this with reference to the blood pH, concentration of carbon dioxide, and oxygen.

CHAPTER FIVE

Oxygen and carbon dioxide transport

How are oxygen and carbon dioxide carried in the blood? Does the supply of oxygen and the removal of carbon dioxide limit performance? Can the transport of these gases be improved in any way, and how? What is the effect of training on the blood gas transport systems? Why is it impossible to work as hard at high altitudes as at sea level?

In exercise, the metabolic rate can rise from a resting oxygen consumption of 250 ml/min to a maximum value of 4000 ml/min (for an active young man). This sixteen-fold increase in demand must be catered for by just a five-fold change in cardiac output. Clearly, the quantity of oxygen delivered by the blood flow must improve considerably to balance the equation. Changes in the efficiency of oxygen delivery are intimately related to the increase in cardiac output, its distribution within the body, and to the oxygen demand of the tissues.

Oxygen transport requires haemoglobin

Oxygen is not particularly readily dissolved in water. At the temperature of arterial blood, one litre of water exposed to atmospheric air dissolves less than 5 ml of oxygen (Fig. 5.1). On the other hand, at rest the body needs to be supplied with 250 ml of oxygen each minute. If blood contained only plasma, at least 50 litres (11 gallons) would have to be pumped around the body each minute to supply our resting oxygen requirement! Since this is twice as much as the cardiovascular system can deliver, even at full stretch (Ch. 6), it is clear that a special oxygen transport mechanism must be involved.

This special mechanism is the iron-rich protein, haemoglobin, which gives blood its red colour. Haemoglobin combines reversibly with oxygen where the gas is abundant, and gives it up readily where oxygen is in poor supply. Haemoglobin has been a success-

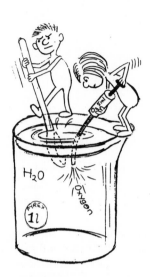
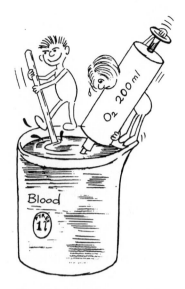

Fig. 5.1 Oxygen is not very water soluble, holding only 0.5% of its own volume of the gas in solution at body temperatures.

Fig. 5.2 Thanks to its haemoglobin content, blood holds 20% of its own volume of oxygen in solution.

ful and popular device for oxygen carriage for over 1000 million years. Virtually all vertebrates have adopted it, as have some invertebrates. With minor changes to the molecule, evolution has tailored haemoglobin to suit the needs of a wide variety of animals and environments, ranging from cold-blooded fish and iguanas to warm-blooded whales and camels, from sea level rats and horses to high altitude guinea pigs and llamas.

Each haemoglobin molecule combines with four oxygen molecules, or one gram of haemoglobin binds with 1.4 ml of oxygen. Since each litre of blood contains 150 grams of haemoglobin, the maximum oxygen carrying capacity of blood is just over 200 ml of oxygen per litre of blood (Fig. 5.2). This is fifty times the oxygen carrying capacity of plasma. Accordingly, we need far less blood to deliver oxygen than would be required if the cardiovascular system was filled with plasma.

Haemoglobin is a small protein, and if it was simply dissolved in plasma, the kidney would filter it out of the body and lose it in

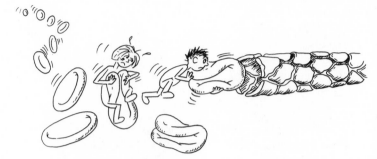

Fig. 5.3 Haemoglobin is carried in specialised cells called red-cells which are a tight fit in the smallest capillaries.

the urine. Instead, haemoglobin is packed into red cells. (In certain diseases where red cells are damaged, haemoglobin appears in urine, darkening it, eg Blackwater Fever, or terminal malaria.) In addition, packing haemoglobin into red cells gives blood a lower viscosity than it would have if the pigment was dissolved directly in the plasma.

Red cells begin life with a collection of all the usual sub-microscopic organelles (nucleus, mitochondria, etc.) which most cells have. As they mature, these organelles are lost, leaving the maximum amount of space for haemoglobin inside. The cells also develop a flattish "biconcave" shape (Fig. 5.3) giving them a large surface area to assist diffusion. They are so flexible that they bend readily to pass through the capillaries, and need to since many capillaries are smaller than red cells. Bending also forces the red cells up against the walls of the capillaries, ensuring that the distance the oxygen must travel between the red cell and its destination is kept as short as possible.

Oxygen transport in the blood

The amount of oxygen carried by haemoglobin depends upon the partial pressure (the proportion of total gas pressure which can be assigned to each component of a mixture) of the gas to which it is exposed. The atmospheric pressure is 760 mmHg. Since the atmosphere is 79% nitrogen and 21% oxygen, the partial pressure of oxygen in the atmosphere is 21% of 760, or 160 mmHg. In the lungs, since oxygen is continually removed, its partial pressure drops to about 100 mmHg or about 13% of the lung gas. This is

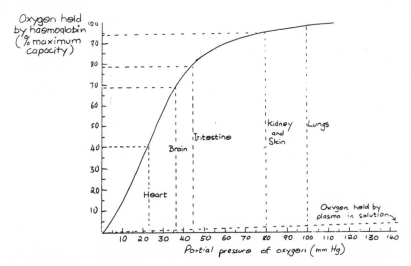

Fig. 5.4 *Haemoglobin combines reversibly with oxygen. If the partial pressure of oxygen is high (as in the lungs) haemoglobin takes up oxygen. In tissues which have high metabolic rates, the local partial pressure is low and haemoglobin gives up oxygen to the tissue.*

the maximum oxygen concentration found in the body. In all other tissues, since they use oxygen, the partial pressure is lower. The lowest oxygen partial pressures are found in the blood leaving hard working muscle, where they can be as low as 10 mmHg.

It is worth emphasising that the oxygen content of blood and its partial pressure in blood are very different things. Thus, in anaemia the haemoglobin content of blood is low, and the amount of oxygen which can be carried is also low, even though the partial pressure of oxygen may be normal. Likewise, in carbon monoxide poisoning, some of the blood's haemoglobin is strongly attached to carbon monoxide reducing the amount of haemoglobin available to carry oxygen. Here, the victim may die of oxygen lack even with plenty available in the lungs. Note that the amount of oxygen dissolved in the plasma is very small (Figs. 5.1 & 5.4).

The most effective treatment for carbon monoxide poisoning requires several hours in a hyperbaric (high pressure) chamber filled with oxygen. Under high pressure, oxygen is able to drive carbon monoxide away from haemoglobin despite their close attachment. Anti-pollution regulations have so reduced carbon monoxide emissions from cars that carbon monoxide poisoning has become rare. The replacement of coal gas with natural gas has also helped!

The higher the oxygen partial pressure, the more oxygen will attach itself to haemoglobin, until all the positions or sites for attachment are full, and the haemoglobin molecule is said to be saturated. The relationship between oxygen partial pressure and oxygen binding onto haemoglobin is complex (Fig. 5.4). At the usual oxygen partial pressure found in the lungs, haemoglobin is 98% saturated with oxygen. That is, nearly every haemoglobin molecule has combined with four oxygen molecules, and each litre of normal blood contains about 200 ml of oxygen. This oxygen-ated blood is pumped around the body in the arteries to satisfy the needs of metabolism.

Haemoglobin loses its oxygen in oxygen poor environments. The amount of oxygen unloaded is proportional to the oxygen partial pressure in the tissue through which the blood is flowing (Fig. 5.4). Since they use oxygen, all of the body's tissues have lower oxygen partial pressures than arterial blood. Organs with high metabolic rates tend to have low oxygen partial pressures. Thus, when arterial blood passes through a particularly active tissue, it gives up more oxygen than it does travelling through a resting tissue. Figure 5.4 shows the partial pressures and corres-ponding oxygen contents of blood leaving various organs.

Factors other than the local oxygen content affect the binding of oxygen to haemoglobin. In an acid medium, haemoglobin unloads more oxygen (Fig. 5.5). High temperature also promotes oxygen loss. Conditions tend to be acidic in regions with a high metabolic rate due to the high rate of carbon dioxide (which forms carbonic acid in solution) production. A high rate of metabolism also raises the temperature. Both of these conditions favour the release of oxygen, and assist oxygen delivery. Figure 5.4 gives examples of oxygen extraction by several tissues. Thus the kidney, which re-ceives a generous blood flow relative to its metabolic rate, removes only 8% of the oxygen supplied to it, while the resting heart with a low blood flow relative to its metabolic rate removes 60% of the available oxygen.

Oxygen delivery in muscle

Not all of the oxygen bound to haemoglobin can be removed in the tissues. The only way in which all of the oxygen could be removed from blood would be to reduce the local partial pressure of the gas to zero. If this were to occur, the chemical reactions of

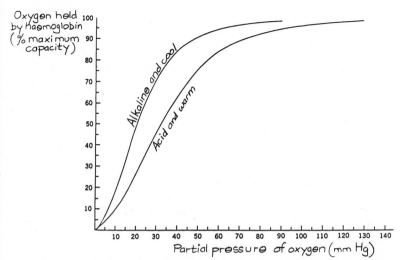

Fig. 5.5 The ability of haemoglobin to combine with oxygen also de-pends on the temperature and the acidity of the environment. Working muscle is hot and acid, and picks up more oxygen than expected from blood. In the lungs, conditions are cool and alkaline, encouraging haemo-globin to load up with oxygen.

metabolism would stop for lack of oxygen and the tissue would die. Tissues must have oxygen supplied at a rate which matches their metabolic requirement, and to maintain an oxygen concentration (or partial pressure) high enough to allow metabolism to operate.

The oxygen concentration within cells is difficult to gauge. It is very low in the mitochondria of hard working muscle. Some scientists have estimated that this partial pressure may be less than 1% of the value in atmospheric air. The partial pressure of oxygen in the venous blood draining a tissue is easier to measure and can be taken as an index of the abundance of oxygen within the tissue. As judged by the oxygen partial pressure in their venous blood, organs differ greatly in their ability to extract oxygen from arterial blood. This depends on several factors, such as the rate at which oxygen is used by the tissue, the distance between the cell and its nearest capillary, the speed of flow through (or the time blood is in contact with) the tissue, and the general environment the tissue presents to the blood (temperature and acidity).

Blood flows swiftly through the kidney and in large volume because the kidney's job is to regulate blood composition and to excrete waste products. Accordingly, blood leaves the kidney with most of its original oxygen content and with a partial pressure of around 60 mmHg. The brain removes only 30% of the oxygen delivered to it, and the partial pressure of oxygen in the blood leaving the brain is 35 mmHg (Fig. 5.4). At the other extreme, working skeletal muscle may remove more than 80% of the oxygen it receives, corresponding to a venous oxygen partial pressure of around 15 mmHg. The ability of exercising muscle to remove oxygen from blood is due to a combination of its high temperature, its acidity, and to its rich blood supply which ensures that no cell is very far from a blood-filled capillary. However, even more important is the relative oxygen deprivation which is forced on muscle.

During exercise, vasoconstrictor nerve signals are received by all tissues requiring them to accept a lower rate of blood flow than they would "like to have" (p. 135). This, in turn lowers their oxygen partial pressure forcing them to extract more of the gas from the blood supply. Since the cardiac output is limited to just a five-fold increase from rest to exercise, while the metabolic rate increases sixteen-fold, improved oxygen extraction is a vital part of the cardiovascular system's capacity to adequately support activity.

Working muscle can remove more oxygen from its blood supply than any other tissue. But how can muscle tolerate the very low oxygen concentration required to achieve this? In all probability individual muscle cells experience a minimum oxygen concentration which is not very different from that which, for example, the brain experiences. However, nerve cells in the brain do not contact their blood supply directly because a layer of protective glial cells surrounds them. On the other hand, muscle has a very high density of capillaries which brings each cell very close to its oxygen supply. Muscle also has a high tolerance to acid so that the high concentrations of carbon dioxide caused by exercise do not harm muscle, and even assist oxygen delivery. By comparison, brain tissue is intolerant of acid and requires a brisk blood flow to keep its surroundings refreshed.

Another factor is the red pigment, myoglobin, which is present in muscle. Myoglobin is related to haemoglobin and oxygen also

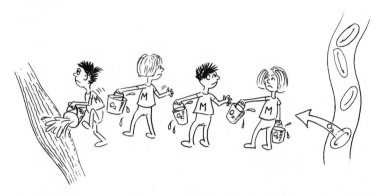

Fig. 5.6 Myoglobin combines reversibly with oxygen in a manner similar to haemoglobin. It is present, particularly in slow twitch muscle (Ch. 2), where it enhances oxygen diffusion.

binds to it. Myoglobin's purpose, however, is not to store oxygen. Rather, myoglobin improves the solubility of oxygen in muscle tissue. This increase in solubility has the effect of speeding the rate of oxygen diffusion through muscle, and of increasing the oxygen concentration at the muscle cell. The concentration of myoglobin is greatest in aerobic or slow twitch muscles which can have very high rates of oxygen consumption. Their high myoglobin content gives them a dark colour. On the other hand, anaerobic or fast twitch muscle has far less myoglobin and tends to be pale (see p. 17). (Slow twitch muscle also has a generous blood supply which darkens it relative to fast twitch muscle.)

Carbon dioxide transport in blood

Unlike oxygen, carbon dioxide is very soluble in water. The partial pressure of carbon dioxide in the lung is less than half that of oxygen, and yet each litre of blood carries over half a litre of carbon dioxide. This is nearly three times the amount of oxygen which blood can carry, even with the help of haemoglobin.

Carrying oxygen in blood causes no change in the pH (acidity). However, when carbon dioxide is dissolved in water, it forms carbonic acid. (In blood this happens rapidly with the help of an enzyme present in the red cell.) The loss of carbon dioxide in the lungs reduces the acidity of the blood, while its production in

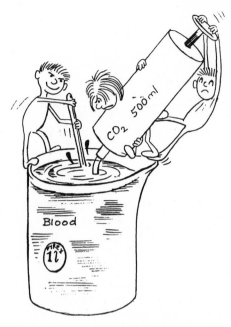

Fig. 5.7 Carbon dioxide is very soluble in either water or blood. Blood will hold half its volume of carbon dioxide in solution. (Compare this with Fig. 5.2)

various tissues increases acidity. Changes in the acidity of the blood are undesirable, and are minimised in several ways.

While there is a limit to the amount of oxygen which haemoglobin can carry, there is none to the amount of carbon dioxide which can dissolve in blood. This depends only on the local partial pressure of carbon dioxide, and by a tissue's ability to tolerate the acidity produced when the gas is dissolved. Thus, muscle tolerates acidity well while the brain does not.

The blood is well buffered against changes in pH. A buffer is a dissolved substance which combines with acid, neutralising it. There are several buffers in blood. One is dissolved sodium bicarbonate (baking soda). Haemoglobin is an important buffer which actually becomes more effective as it loses oxygen — which conveniently occurs just where carbon dioxide is produced. The plasma proteins, which bind carbon dioxide loosely, also act as buffers.

As blood passes through the lungs, only about 50 ml of carbon dioxide are removed from each litre, or just 10% of the total dissolved. Having a large total amount in solution and adding or removing only a small proportion of this helps to minimise changes in blood pH. It is worth bearing in mind that control of the amount of carbon dioxide in the arterial blood is the body's most important short term means of regulating pH. An example of how this works in an emergency (at high rates of anaerobic work) can be seen in Ch. 4.

Is the supply of oxygen limiting in exercise?

The cardiovascular system's ability to supply oxygen probably limits the amount of aerobic work which can be performed. For example, oxygen availability is reduced at high altitude. If a particular work load is first performed at sea level and then repeated at high altitude, the cardiac output is lower during the sea level trial since the smaller amount of blood is able to carry enough oxygen to satisfy demand. In an all-out effort at high altitude, the maximum oxygen consumption and the amount of work which can be done are substantially reduced compared to the sea level values. This reduction is proportional to the oxygen content of the arterial blood, and suggests that the cardiovascular system has no spare capacity available to compensate for the lack of oxygen at high altitudes.

The maximum oxygen consumption in treadmill running can be increased by 10–12% if the subjects breathe 50% oxygen in nitrogen instead of air (21% oxygen). Cardiac output is similar in both cases. Since the oxygen use and the work output respond to the slight increase in oxygen carrying capacity, this suggests that aerobic metabolism is indeed limited by the oxygen supply.

Studies have been performed on subjects pedalling an exercise bicycle first with the right leg and then with both legs. During both tests, the oxygen consumption of the right leg was measured. When the left leg was made to work as well, cardiac output increased, but did not double. This reduced the amount of oxygen available to the right leg, and its rate of oxygen utilisation was also reduced.

Thus, there is good evidence that oxygen utilisation and aerobic work output are limited by the oxygen supply to muscle. This, of

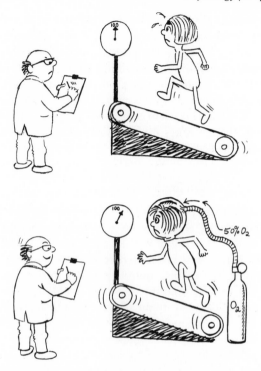

Fig. 5.8 Breathing oxygen slightly improves performance, but at some cost in mobility. (Also refer to Ch. 9, p. 215).

course, points to the cardiovascular system being the limiting factor in aerobic performance.

The oxygen delivery system responds to endurance training. This subject is dealt with in Ch. 6.

high altitude training

Some 10–15 years ago, a group of athletes emerged from various high altitude villages in Kenya, Tanzania and Ethiopia to win endurance races at the Mexico City Olympics. Since Mexico City is 7000 ft (2000 m) above sea level, for some time it became fashionable to train for endurance athletics at a high altitude location.

One response to high altitude hypoxia is that new capillaries develop in muscle, increasing the density of the blood supply and reducing the diffusion distance. The concentration of the enzymes which are responsible for aerobic metabolism also increases, tending to improve oxygen uptake. Finally, high altitude hypoxia stimulates the production of red cells, raising the red cell and haemoglobin content of the blood within a few weeks. This increases its oxygen carrying capacity — but also increases blood viscosity, thus tending to reduce the cardiac output. Occasionally, natives of high altitude develop a disease (Monge's Disease) in which red cells form over 75% of the blood volume (45% is normal), more than doubling the blood viscosity.

Several weeks of training at high altitude can make sea level athletes competitive with mountain natives at high altitude athletic meetings. However, there is little evidence that a period of training at high altitude similarly benefits athletes who then compete at sea level. The likely reason for this is that both oxygen consumption and the work output are limited at high altitude. It may be that the reduced intensity of training which can be carried out in a high altitude training programme may result in a slight "detraining" effect, counteracting any increase in oxygen carrying capacity.

Another explanation may be that high altitude training reduces the amount of bicarbonate buffer in blood (see p. 79). This, in turn, may make the athlete less able to cope with the high concentrations of lactic acid which occur in competitive athletic events. However, the normal bicarbonate content of the blood, and its buffering capacity, is usually restored within 24 hours, making this an unlikely explanation.

Finally, endurance is often limited by the combined effects of reduced blood volume and increased blood viscosity as water (sweat) is lost from the body (Ch. 8). High altitude training increases the concentration of red cells in the blood. Thus, altitude trained athletes' blood viscosity starts high, and gets higher still as water is lost (see p. 181).

blood doping

If the oxygen supply limits exercise, then increasing the cardiovascular system's ability to deliver oxygen should improve performance. Well trained endurance athletes, have already achieved much of this by increasing both the density of capillaries in muscle and their cardiac output. However, endurance training causes a larger increase in plasma volume than in red cell volume. Thus, the

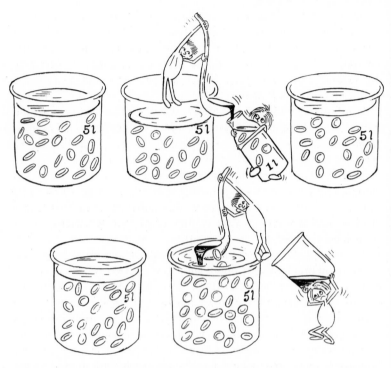

Fig. 5.9 Blood is 45% red cells. In blood doping, one litre of blood is removed and the 450 ml of red cells are stored. The remaining blood has reduced volume but normal cell concentration. In a day or two, blood volume is restored, but the concentration of red cells is now 36% — a mild anaemia. After one month both blood volume and red cell concentration are normal. In storage, some red cells disintegrate. Say 400 ml of red cells are reinfused. The total volume is now 5.4 litres and the concentration of red cells is 49%. Oxygen carrying capacity is improved for 2–3 weeks.

blood of endurance trained athletes is slightly "thin", and has a lower than normal concentration of red cells.

Athletes, always diligent in their search for maximum performance, have noted this blood thinning and tried to improve their oxygen carring capacity. This is done by "blood doping" in which an athlete removes and stores about a litre of blood at least one month before an important event. All of the blood volume and most of the lost cells are replaced by the time of competition. The stored red cells (the normal lifespan of red cells is 90 days, and depending on the storage method, some disintegrate in storage) are re-infused on the day of the event, markedly increasing the oxygen carrying capacity of the blood. The added red cells survive for several weeks in the circulation, so that any effect seen should continue for a week or two.

Reinfusion of 400 ml of red cells increases the oxygen-carrying capacity by about 16%. However, any resulting increase in maximum oxygen consumption is variable, and may even be absent. Average figures of 5−15% have been reported by different researchers. Since the red cells contribute to blood viscosity, blood doping increases viscosity, reducing both the maximum heart rate and cardiac output. Which effect should dominate in any individual — increased oxygen carriage, or reduced cardiac performance — is hard to predict.

Accordingly, the results of actual trials of blood doping vary. Some report no effect on performance, while others claim gains in both endurance and speed. In the "1/100 second" world of the athlete, any potential improvement, however small, may mean the difference between first and fourth place and be worth any effort to secure. Also, there are no studies which suggest that blood doping might worsen performance. That seems to make it a "one-way bet". Since the procedure is not detectable with any certainty, despite being banned, it is probably widely used.

On theoretical grounds, blood doping may offer advantages in middle distance races. Increases in blood viscosity caused by the loss of sweat become important after an hour of strenuous activity (Ch. 8), and if viscosity has already been increased by blood doping, performance would probably be adversely affected in events like the marathon or the Tour de France.

The advantages of blood doping — if any — may not be due to an improvement in oxygen transport. Rather, the period of time before re-infusion, during which the athlete has trained with blood having a lower than normal oxygen carrying capacity, may be responsible. This may mimic some of the effects of high altitude exposure by reducing the availability of oxygen (see above).

Another explanation of the effects of blood doping is psychological. Thus, an athlete who thinks that he/she has gained an advantage over their competitors by means of this technique may acquire the extra self-confidence to put in a better performance.

Summary

In summary, it is likely that the cardiovascular system's ability to deliver oxygen may limit athletic performance. Reinfusion of an athletes own red cells always increases the oxygen carrying capacity of blood. This is often translated into an increase in maximum oxygen uptake by the athlete, and may result in either improved speed or endurance or both. Training at high altitude also increases the number of red cells and the oxygen carrying capacity of blood. This improves athletic performance in a high altitude environment — but not to sea level standards. However, high altitude training seldom improves sea level performance, making it less clear exactly how blood doping may work.

Blood doping is illegal. It is also unsporting since its (arguable) advantages are only available to those competitors who are wealthy or lucky enough to have access to an unscrupulous doctor. There is some danger involved since hygienic facilities to remove and store blood for long periods of time and to separate cells from plasma must be available. It is, of course, futile to suggest that athletes with access to such facilities should refrain from taking advantage of them in order to ensure a fair contest — there is simply too much money and fame at stake in today's world of sports competition (Ch. 9).

CHAPTER SIX

The cardiovascular system

Part 1 — Cardiovascular physiology

The central purpose of the cardiovascular system is to move substances around the body. These are the materials and waste products involved in metabolism. Foodstuffs such as glucose and fatty acids, and reagents such as oxygen are brought to tissues via the blood stream, while wastes such as carbon dioxide and heat are removed.

In addition to its transport function, the cardiovascular system supplies hydraulic power to certain organs. Thus, blood pressure powers the kidney's filtration of the blood and inflates erectile tissue.

Control of the cardiovascular system is exercised with a view to its transport function. The system's performance is gauged by whether the body's organs are "satisfied" with their blood supply and the rate at which materials are delivered and removed. The system's performance is also constantly adjusted to minimise the amount of work the heart has to perform.

Functional anatomy

The cardiovascular system consists of certain basic elements: (1) a working fluid (the blood) which transports materials around the body, (2) a pump to move the blood, (3) some plumbing to carry the flow, (4) special porous plumbing where blood is brought into close contact with tissues so that substances may pass (or exchange) between the blood and the cells, and (5) control mechanisms which ensure the efficient operation of the system.

1. *The blood volume.* Blood is the fluid within the cardiovascular system whose main job is to transport substances around the body, particularly oxygen and carbon dioxide (Ch. 5). Its volume is approximately 5 litres (in a 70 kg man) or 3.5 litres (in

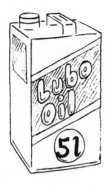

Fig. 6.1

a 60 kg woman). The volume of the pulmonary (lung) circuit is 9% of the total while the systemic circuit contains 84%. The rest is the volume of the heart, about 350 ml or 7%.

2. *Pump.* The heart is the main pump of the cardiovascular system. It provides the energy to pressurise the system, and to circulate blood around the body. There is also a diffusely located secondary pump which uses the body's muscles for power — muscle contraction squeezes veins passing through them and, with the help of valves, promotes the return of blood to the heart.

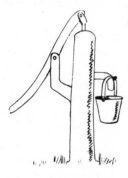

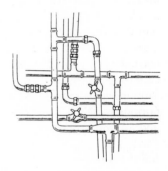

Fig. 6.2   Fig. 6.3

3. *Plumbing.* The heart is connected to a system of tubing which guides blood flow around the body. The arteries are thick-walled and take high pressure blood away from the heart. The veins are thin-walled and return low pressure blood to the heart. However, this tubing is not passive like normal plumbing, but changes its shape and size. In so doing, arteries and veins play an important role in controlling the performance of the cardiovascular system.

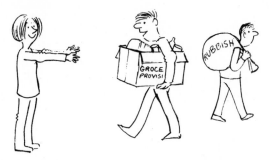

Fig. 6.4

4. *Exchange.* Once blood has arrived in an organ, substances must be delivered to the tissue and waste material removed. This exchange is carried out in the capillaries which are very small, thin-walled, porous vessels so widely distributed around the body that no cell is far from one. Diffusion is the main means by which substances move the short distance separating a cell from its neighbouring capillary. Over such small distances, diffusion is a rapid and efficient means of exchange.

5. *Control.* The cardiovascular system is equipped with control mechanisms. These consist of sensing devices which monitor cardiovascular performance, a computer which digests this information and issues commands in the form of nervous and hormonal signals, and the muscles of the heart, arteries, veins, and accessory systems which obey these instructions.

6. *Form or actual anatomy.* These elements are arranged in the following manner: There are two separate circuits, each with its own pump and vessels. The right side of the heart receives oxygen depleted blood from the body and pumps it to the lungs. This is the pulmonary circulation. The left side of the heart receives oxygenated blood from the lungs and pumps it to the rest of the body. This is the systemic circulation.

The arteries, after repeated branching, deliver blood to the capillary vessels in both circuits where exchange occurs. From the capillaries blood is returned to the heart via the veins. The capillaries are so arranged that blood travels through only one capillary bed before returning to the heart. There are three cases where blood flows through two capillary beds one after

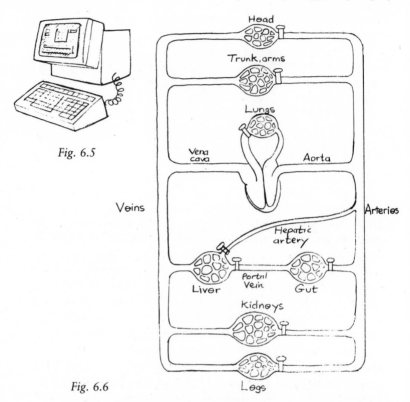

Fig. 6.5

Fig. 6.6

the other: the liver receives venous blood from the digestive tract as well as its own arterial supply; within the kidney blood flows through two capillary beds in series; and the pituitary gland receives venous blood from the base of the brain. With those exceptions, every tissue receives freshly oxygenated blood under adequate pressure.

Blood flow in tubes

Fluid flows when pressure is applied to it. Fluids have viscosity and there is friction between the fluid and the vessel wall. These cause resistance, and flow can be calculated:

$$\text{FLOW} = \frac{(\text{PRESSURE})\,(\text{RADIUS})^4}{(\text{LENGTH})\,(\text{VISCOSITY})} \times \frac{\pi}{8}$$

The rate of flow is directly proportional to pressure, but inversely proportional to blood viscosity and to tubing length. However, viscosity and length normally remain constant. Note particularly that small changes in the size of the blood vessels (radius) have a large effect on flow. Thus, a 19% increase in radius doubles flow. Changes in the radius of blood vessels are the most important means by which blood flow through a tissue is controlled.

The heart — self-excitation

The heart is a pump made entirely of rhythmically contracting muscle. It is (like most of the body's organs) a very reliable device, beating over 100,000 times per day, or about 40,000,000 times a year. In the majority of people, the heart is still working after 70 years and more than 3 billion beats.

Most of the body's muscles must be told to contract. In the absence of such instruction, they remain relaxed. Fortunately, we do not need to remember to stimulate the heart (nor can we stop it) since it is self-exciting and initiates its own beat. If removed from the body, the heart would continue to contract rhythmically for as long as it is oxygenated, fed, and kept warm. Each cell within the heart is potentially self-exciting.

All cells carry a small voltage or potential across their membranes so that the inside of the cell is negative with respect to the outside (see p. 8). Some cells respond when stimulated and are called "excitable". These include muscle, nerve, and some glandular tissue. One type of stimulus is a small electrical shock, large enough to reduce the cell's resting membrane potential to a threshold value, stimulating it. In heart muscle, the resting potential is not stable, but spontaneously "leaks" away. When it drops to a threshold value, the cell is stimulated, reversing the voltage inside the cell to a positive value. This "action potential" activates the mechanisms causing muscle contraction (see p. 11). Following contraction, the resting membrane potential is restored, and the process repeats itself.

Most of the body's muscle cells are separate from each other and act independently. However, the cells in heart muscle are all electrically connected to each other. Stimulation of one cell results in the spread of excitation throughout the heart muscle, and the heart's contraction as a unit.

If a heart were cut into small pieces and placed in a warm, oxygenated nutrient solution, each piece would continue to excite itself and contract. Different regions of the heart have a characteristic rate at which they contract. Ventricular muscle is slowest at around thirty beats per minute, while atrial muscle is faster. A small region of the right atrium, the pacemaker, is fastest with a normal rate of self-excitation of around 120 beats per minute.

This pacemaker region (also called the sino-atrial or S-A node) delivers a stimulus to the heart before any other region can recover from the previous beat, and governs the heart rate. However, the heart's resting rate is usually 60–70 beats per minute, and not 120. This is because the pacemaker's natural hurry is braked by nerve signals from the brain telling it to slow down. During sleep, the heart slows further to fifty beats per minute or even less, while removal of the braking signal and adding stimulatory nerve signals to accelerate it can whip the heart to over three beats per second when required.

Initially the pacemaker just stimulates the atrial muscle. The ventricular muscle is insulated from the atrial muscle and cannot be directly stimulated by it. The atrial action potential arrives at the ventricle via a small group of cells lying between the four heart valves, the atrio-ventricular (A-V) node. The A-V node delays the electrical stimulus, allowing atrial contraction to finish before the ventricles begin to contract (Fig. 6.7).

In certain forms of heart disease, the A-V node is damaged and fails to conduct the atrial impulse. This is called heart block, and the pulse rate may drop to thirty per minute (the natural ventricular rythm). At such a slow rate the heart cannot pump enough blood. Heart block patients are treated by the surgical implanta-

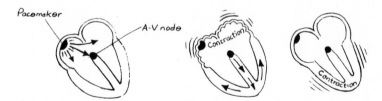

Fig. 6.7 The pacemaker first stimulates the two atria. After a brief delay, the stimulus is passed via the A-V node to the ventricles, which thus contract shortly after the atria.

tion of an electronic pacemaker whose electrodes stimulate the ventricle. Early pacemakers offered only one rate, a compromise between the requirements of rest and activity. More modern ones with two rates were still unable to synchronise atrial and ventricular contractions, reducing the efficiency of pumping, particularly at high rates (p. 127). The most recent pacemakers trigger from the atrial impulse, offering smooth and natural control of the heart rate, plus normal synchronisation of the atrial and ventricular contractions.

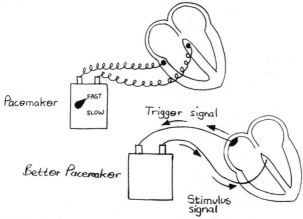

Fig. 6.8 In heart block, artificial pacemakers are implanted to stimulate the ventricles. Older ones have just one or two speeds. If the natural pacemaker is undamaged, the most modern artificial pacemakers amplify its signal and stimulate the ventricles at any rate the body demands.

The electrical activity of cardiac muscle produces small voltages which can be detected by electrodes on the surface of the body and recorded. These recordings are called electrocardiograms or ECGs (sometimes EKG), and certain aspects of the heart's health can be deduced from them.

the heart as a pump
The heart is a double pump — in effect, two separate pumps, the right side delivers blood to the lungs and the left side pumps it to the rest of the body (Fig. 6.9). Each side of the heart is a pump with two stages: a low pressure chamber, the thin walled atrium;

and a high pressure chamber, the much more muscular ventricle. These chambers are separated by valves which ensure that blood flows in the forward direction (Fig. 6.9).

Blood enters the right atrium via the vena cava, and the left atrium via the pulmonary veins. When the atrial muscle contracts its contents are squeezed and the pressure rises. Although the ventricles fill continuously when they are relaxed, atrial contraction briefly increases the rate of filling, topping them up. The ventricles contract just after the atria, closing the atrio-ventricular valves. On the left, contraction raises ventricular pressure until it is higher than the pressure within the aorta. This opens the aortic valve and allows the ventricle to empty. On the right, ventricular pressure must overcome the far lower pulmonary arterial pressure to discharge blood into the circulation of the lungs.

The ventricular contraction is called systole. In a resting individual the pressure developed by the left ventricle during systole is normally 120 mmHg, but only 25 mmHg in the right ventricle (hence the right ventricular muscle is thinner and weaker than the left). Despite the disparity in strength, both pump the same average volume of blood (precisely) per beat. Ventricular relaxation is called diastole, when the pressure in both ventricles drops to zero allowing them to fill from the venous system.

Pressure in the arteries is maintained by the aortic valves on the

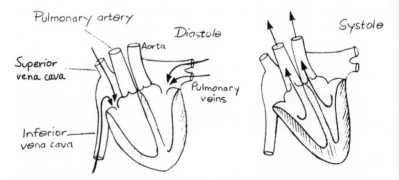

Fig. 6.9 Valves ensure that the heart pumps blood in the forward direction. During diastole the atrio-ventricular valves open admitting blood into the ventricles from the atria. During systole the arterial valves open allowing the ventricles to empty.

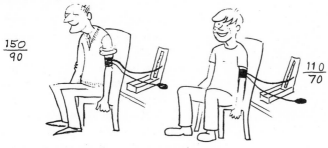

$\dfrac{150}{90}$

$\dfrac{110}{70}$

Fig. 6.10

left, and by the pulmonary arterial valves on the right, preventing blood from flowing back into the heart. Nevertheless, the arterial pressure drops during diastole as blood flows out of the arteries to various tissues. During systole the arteries stretch to receive the volume discharged by the heart, absorbing some of the energy given to the blood during systole. During diastole they give up this energy, stored in their elastic tissue. This helps maintain blood pressure between beats. At rest, the normal diastolic pressure is 80 mmHg in the aorta and 10 mmHg in the pulmonary artery.

The arterial pressure is easy to measure and is given as systolic/ diastolic. The normal value is 120/80, although this varies widely between individuals and through the day. Blood pressure decreases in sleep and increases during stress. With advancing age, blood pressure tends to rise, but mainly in industrial societies. This rise may be due to the environment, since people in underdeveloped countries often maintain a youthfully low blood pressure throughout life. People whose blood pressure is high are said to suffer from hypertension. They are given treatment if their blood pressure exceeds 160/95. High blood pressure places an extra work load on the heart, increases the likelihood of strokes, damages arteries, and accelerates the progress of atherosclerosis.

The structure of blood vessels

Blood vessels are built up of four components (Fig. 6.11). First there is an inner lining of thin endothelial cells. These cells are smooth, slippery and have special properties which prevent the blood from clotting on their walls. The lining allows free diffusion

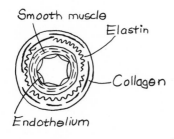

Fig. 6.11

of most substances. However, red blood cells, proteins, and platelets (part of the clotting mechanism) are too large to pass through, and remain in the circulation.

Vascular smooth muscle surrounds the endothelial cell lining. Both the appearance and properties of smooth muscle differ from those of the skeletal muscle which makes our bodies move, and from the heart's cardiac muscle. Contraction of vascular smooth muscle reduces the diameter of a blood vessel, while its relaxation increases it.

Elastin fibres, as their name suggests, are elastic. They are readily stretched by the pressure of blood within the vessel. When elastin is stretched tension is progressively developed, resisting further stretch. Because of this, the diameter of elastic blood vessels is easy to control.

Collagen fibres are made of the same protein material as elastin (with similar proportions of the amino acids which are the building blocks of all proteins), but differently constructed, and very much stiffer. Elastin can be compared to a knitted fabric (Fig. 6.12a) while collagen is like a woven one (Fig. 6.12b). Although chemically quite similar, they have very different properties. Collagen resists stretch serving the same purpose in a blood vessel as the cord in a pneumatic tyre casing. It prevents shape distortion and blowout under pressure.

Types of blood vessels

Blood vessels have different functions and are purpose built in different sizes and with varying proportions of the four basic components (Fig. 6.13).

large arteries

Large arteries contain a great deal of elastin and collagen. They stretch readily, but also resist tearing under high pressure. They have relatively little muscle, hence a limited ability to alter their diameter and blood flow.

Arteries stretch to receive the output of the heart, absorbing and

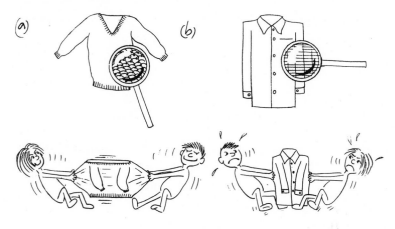

Fig. 6.12

storing some of the energy the heart has put into the arterial blood. This willingness to stretch limits the rise in pressure during each systole. Between beats (diastole) the elastic material in the arteries returns this stored energy to the blood flow, maintaining the pressure. The large arteries act as pressure reservoirs, smoothing the pulsatile output of the heart (pressure 120/0) into the steadier pressure characteristic of arteries (120/80).

In old age, the arteries become stiff resulting in high systolic pressures. In "hardening of the arteries", when stiffness increases substantially, much of the smoothing function is lost, producing a combination of high systolic and low diastolic pressures (eg 200/60).

arterioles
Arterioles are very small arteries with an internal diameter (0.04 mm) only slightly larger than a red blood cell. They are very muscular with a wall thickness similar to their diameter. They have some elastin and collagen, but far less than the larger arteries.

The arterioles' main task is to control local blood flow, which they accomplish by contracting or relaxing their smooth muscle. This changes their radius which has a large effect on vascular resistance (p. 106). Arterioles are responsible for over half of the vascular system's resistance to flow.

pre-capillary sphincters
Pre-capillary sphincters are similar to arterioles, but contain very little elastin. Their lack of elasticity makes them unstable so that muscular

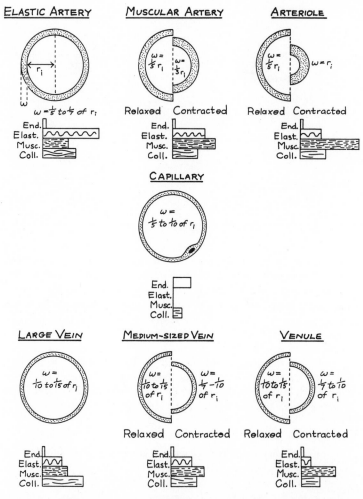

Fig. 6.13 All blood vessels are built up of the same materials: Elastin (Elast.); Collagen (Coll.); Muscle (Musc.); and lined with Endothelial cells (End.). The relative wall thickness (w) and vessel radius (r) are indicated. Medium and small arteries and veins can contract and the degree to which they do is shown. Note that the very small arteries (arterioles) which have a great deal of muscle can contract until their internal radius is similar to their wall thickness.

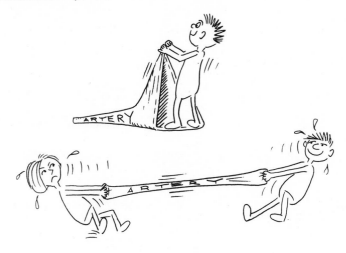

Fig. 6.14

contraction closes them completely while relaxation opens them completely (see elastin, p. 112). They serve much the same purpose as arterioles, but control local blood flow more crudely, periodically switching it on and off.

capillaries

Capillaries are very thin-walled, consisting of just a single layer of epithelial cells. Their internal diameter is often smaller than that of the red blood cells (0.008 mm), which have to bend double to pass through (they bend readily!). Capillaries are leaky, allowing water, salts and certain other dissolved materials to pass through freely. However, larger solutes such as proteins cannot penetrate capillaries. As fluid leaks out of the capillaries, the protein inside becomes more concentrated and the osmotic pressure this creates limits the amount of leakage (Fig. 8.4). (In bruising, capillaries are damaged, allowing protein to leak out and causing oedema or swelling.)

Capillaries allow material to be exchanged between the blood and the tissues through which it flows. Most of this exchange is carried out by diffusion.

venules and veins

Venules are the venous counterpart of arterioles, but their function is similar to that of larger veins. Veins and venules are relatively thin

E

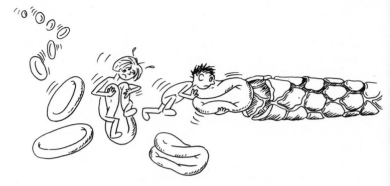

Fig. 6.15 Fortunately, red blood cells are very flexible because the smallest blood vessels can only accommodate them bent double!

walled but their walls are muscular and capable of considerable contraction, although only against the low pressures encountered in the venous circulation. Veins contain elastic and collagenous tissue as well.

About 75% of the blood volume is contained in the venous system, and its main function is to serve as a reservoir. Veins are normally oval in cross-section and readily accept additional fluid with virtually no change in pressure simply by rounding up. Contracting, they can increase venous pressure, and speed the return of blood to the heart.

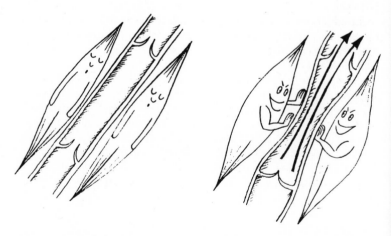

Fig. 6.16 Muscle contraction "massages" the veins, and returns blood to the heart.

The veins also have valves which ensure that blood flows only in the forward direction. External pressure on a vein causes the blood within it to flow towards the heart. Such pressure may be applied by limb muscles contracting around veins, and the resulting flow is important in assisting the return of blood to the heart during exercise.

The heart — performance

output
The performance of the heart can be gauged in various ways. Its ability to pump blood is probably most important. The heart relies on changes in both the rate and in the volume of each stroke to alter its output. Thus:

CARDIAC OUTPUT = STROKE VOLUME × HEART RATE

In the average 70 kg (11 st) man each beat of the "resting" ventricle moves 70 ml of blood. At the usual resting rate of 72 beats per minute, each ventricle pumps five litres, or over a gallon of blood per minute. Together, both ventricles pump over fifteen tons of blood each day, equivalent to the volume of a fuel tanker!

As mentioned above, the heart rate at rest is constantly slowed by inhibitory nerve signals to seventy beats per minute. During physical activity this braking is released to speed the heart. If required, stimulatory nerve signals can be applied to accelerate it further. Maximum performance of the heart will be covered in Part 2 of this chapter.

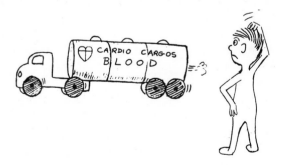

Fig. 6.17 Daily, both sides of the heart together pump about the volume contained in a tank truck.

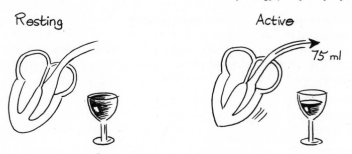

Fig. 6.18 Each ventricle contains approximately the volume of a full wine glass and pumps about half of this during systole.

The amount of blood pumped per beat can also be changed. Normally, at rest each ventricle contains about 150 ml of blood. Each resting heart beat empties about half of this into the appropriate artery (Fig. 6.18). To increase the stroke volume, the strength of contraction must increase to allow more rapid and complete emptying. This is accomplished by the action of adrenaline released into the blood from the adrenal gland, and by noradrenaline from stimulatory nerves released directly into the heart muscle.

Of course the heart cannot pump more blood than it receives, and any increase in output must be exactly matched by an increase in the volume of blood returning to the heart. Another measure of performance is the work accomplished by the heart. This work is determined by both the volume of blood pumped per minute, and by the pressure at which blood is discharged into the arteries.

blood pressure
In order to induce blood to circulate within the cardiovascular system, pressure must be applied to it. This pressure is generated by the action of the heart pumping blood into the arteries, and is directly proportional to the volume of blood pumped (cardiac output) and to the resistance of the circulatory system to its flow:

BLOOD PRESSURE = CARDIAC OUTPUT ×
PERIPHERAL RESISTANCE

Thus, if the output of the heart increases, pressure will rise unless vascular resistance is reduced to compensate. Although blood pressure could be regulated by changes in either resistance or output, resistance is usually adjusted to control pressure.

The blood pressure is well regulated. If the pressure should fall, blood flow through various organs would also fall and their function suffer. The brain is particularly sensitive to the rate of blood flow because it is incapable of anaerobic (without oxygen) metabolism, and most of the devices which monitor arterial blood pressure (the baroreceptors) are located in the arteries which supply the brain.

When the baroreceptors detect falling pressure they inform the brain, which acts quickly to constrict arteries serving relatively less important tissues (intestines, skin, etc.). This increases the vascular resistance. Meanwhile, the output of the heart, and (of course) the rate at which blood returns to the heart are also increased. These manoeuvres tend to restore blood pressure.

The giraffe's blood pressure, measured at the heart, is over double the human value. However, measured at the brain, the giraffe's pressure is similar to ours. In the giraffe, the heart has to overcome the weight of a 10 ft column of blood above the heart before it can begin to supply a flow of blood to the brain, hence its

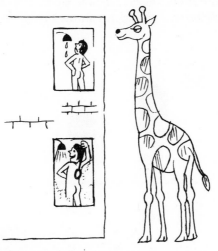

Fig. 6.19 The cardiovascular system's flow control is far more sophisticated than that usually found in homes. Thus, the requirements of a recently fed digestive system are not permitted to rob the brain of its blood supply.

need for high blood pressure. In man, normal blood pressure appears to be set near the minimum value required to lift blood the 18 inches from the heart to the head and then to provide adequate flow through the brain. In tall animals, the blood pressure must set at correspondingly higher values.

The brain's high location ensures that it is the first organ to suffer if blood pressure falls. This is similar to the problem suffered by a person taking a shower on the top floor while somebody flushes a toilet on the floor below — a scalding by the sudden decrease in cold water pressure. The brain has a simple and dramatic method of defending its blood supply in an emergency. If the blood pressure drops, the blood flow to the brain falls. The brain rapidly runs out of oxygen and stops functioning. This causes the person to assume the prone position, restoring the brain's blood flow, at the expense of pride! Normally the blood pressure is accurately and rapidly regulated so that manoeuvres such as standing up have little effect on it or on the blood supply to the brain.

The kidney also has a vested interest in maintaining blood pressure. It forms urine by filtering blood under pressure. If pressure drops, filtration stops. The kidney causes angiotensin, a hormone-like substance, to appear in the blood. Angiotensin is a

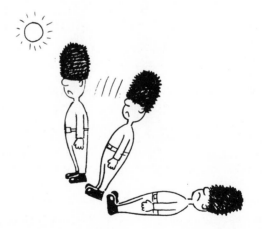

Fig. 6.20 Occasionally the control system fails to maintain blood pressure and blood pressure drops. Fortunately, this is rare and happens only during illness, or when the blood volume has been reduced (eg. by sweating).

powerful stimulant of vascular smooth muscle, constricting blood vessels, and increasing blood pressure. In small animals (rat, mouse), where the effect of gravity is small, blood pressure is similar to the human value. Here, the kidney probably sets the minimum value for blood pressure.

The baroreceptors also keep blood pressure from rising. High blood pressure (hypertension) has a number of harmful effects:

1 increases the work load on the heart
2 encourages development of atherosclerosis
3 damages arteries directly giving rise to strokes
4 causes hypertrophy (overdevelopment) of heart muscle
5 causes stiffening of arterial walls, making hypertension worse.

In hypertension, the control system is disturbed, and no longer maintains a normally low blood pressure. It is not clear whether the fault in the control system has caused the rise in pressure or whether the control system has simply adapted to high pressure caused by some other mechanism.

Cardiovascular control

There are many control systems in the body regulating systems such as the production of digestive juices, the body temperature, and the rate at which water is excreted. The cardiovascular control system is one of the fastest in operation, responding to changes in requirement in seconds.

The cardiovascular system operates to supply the blood flow required by the body under different conditions. Although the flow of blood supplies tissues with many substances and removes many wastes, only two of these are of particular and immediate importance and determine the flow required at any time. One is the supply of oxygen, without which no tissue can long survive. The other is carbon dioxide which dissolves in water to form carbonic acid, accumulation of which severely impairs the chemistry of metabolism.

Cardiovascular regulation is served by two separate control mechanisms: local and central. The system operates under three constraints: (1) maintenance of a relatively constant blood pressure, (2) minimising the work of the heart, and (3) maintenance of a priority blood supply to the brain and the heart.

local control

Local control is a "demand" system in which each tissue demands the blood flow it requires. This is achieved by the simplest possible means. A local increase in metabolic rate raises the concentration of wastes and reduces oxygen. Metabolic wastes (mainly carbon dioxide, plus lactic acid, potassium, adenosine, phosphate, and heat) released within a tissue, plus local oxygen shortage, all relax smooth muscle causing small blood vessels to increase in diameter, lowering resistance. This increases blood flow which, in turn, washes away the wastes and increases the oxygen supply until a new equilibrium is reached.

This local control recognises no limits, nor does it take into account the fact that the heart's ability to pump blood is finite. Limiting regional demand for blood flow and assuring an economical mode of operation for the heart at any level of demand is the task of the central control system.

central control

Central control attempts to moderate and regulate the local demand system. Where local control demands increased flow, central control generally tries to reduce the supply of blood. If a region demands a flow of 750 ml/min, it may receive only 400 ml/min. However, in certain cases central control directs increased blood flow to a specific tissue in the absence of a local demand. One example of this is the increase in blood flow to the skin when the body requires cooling (Ch. 7).

Central control operates by releasing noradrenalin and acetylcholine from nerve endings on blood vessels and by secreting adrenalin from the adrenal gland into the blood stream. Depending on the tissue, these substances may be constrictor, contracting smooth muscle in blood vessels and decreasing blood flow, or dilator, relaxing the smooth muscle and increasing flow. Noradrenalin generally constricts arterioles, while acetylcholine dilates them. Adrenalin is a dilator in most tissues, but also constricts some. (These three substances also affect the strength and frequency of the heart beat, and thus the amount of blood pumped.)

The central control system also ensures that there is an adequate blood flow to the brain and heart, regardless of other demands. This is achieved by maintaining a steady blood pressure in the face of varying flow resistance and changes in the rate at which blood returns to the heart. The brain and heart operate their own de-

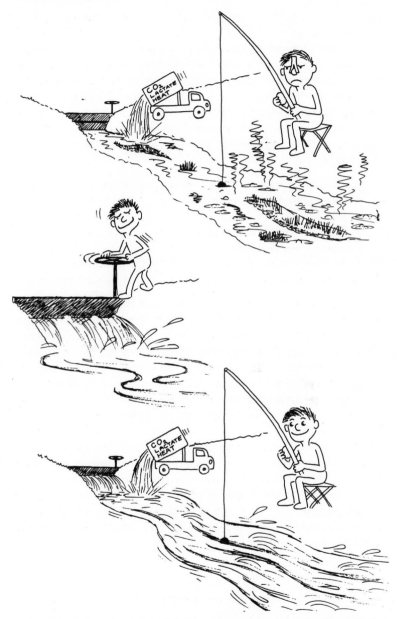

Fig. 6.21 The wastes generated by a tissue cause local "pollution". In response, small blood vessels dilate, increasing flow, and washing away the wastes.

mand systems, but these only work properly if the blood pressure is maintained.

Increased demand for blood flow by a tissue gives rise to a series of cardiovascular adjustments which serve to maintain constant blood pressure. If a tissue dilates its artery and arterioles, the resistance to flow decreases, and the amount of blood passing through them increases. This local fall in resistance reduces the total resistance, and tends to drop blood pressure. The baroreceptors detect the falling pressure and the control system responds in three ways:

1. It attempts to economise by constricting arterioles everywhere (noradrenalin release), reducing flow through other regions.
2. It tells the heart to increase its output (adrenalin and noradrenalin). The heart cannot increase its output unless the amount of blood returning increases.
3. A third response is constriction of the veins increasing venous pressure and augmenting the return flow of blood to the heart.

Central control restrains the demands of the local control systems. If unrestrained, the local blood flow would increase until the concentration of metabolic waste in the tissue became quite low. This would impose a high and unrealistic demand for cardiac output on the heart. By limiting local demand for blood flow the central control system reduces the work load on the heart. This effect becomes more important in exercise when the huge increase in demand would quickly outstrip the pumping ability of the heart.

Central control is also responsible for controlling blood flow in regions which cannot rely on locally generated wastes for automatic demand. Thus, in hot environments, the blood flow to the skin must be increased until it greatly exceeds the metabolic requirement. This flow is required to cool the body. Likewise, the digestive system receives a high blood flow after meals to secrete digestive juices and to absorb foodstuffs, again exceeding the metabolic need.

The effects of haemorrhage; an example of cardiovascular control

Haemorrhage is blood loss. The blood transfusion clinic removes a half litre of blood, or about 10% of the circulating volume. In effect, this is a controlled haemorrhage. The victim of a road accident can lose over two litres of blood, enough to threaten survival. Athletes sometimes have a litre or more of their own blood removed and stored for re-infusion at a later date, hoping to achieve improvements in performance (see p. 99). Finally, sweating removes fluid from the circulation with effects similar to those of haemorrhage.

The loss of a half-litre of blood has little effect and the body's response is hard to detect. On the other hand, the effects of losing two litres of blood are very serious. What are the effects of haemorrhage, and how does the cardiovascular system cope with the blood loss?

The initial result of blood loss is to lower the venous pressure, which reduces the rate at which blood returns to the heart. The ventricles are thus less full at the start of systole, and stroke volume declines. Both the cardiac output and the arterial blood pressure are reduced.

The fall in blood pressure is quickly detected by baroreceptors, and the central control system responds rapidly. Arteries and arterioles around the body constrict, increasing peripheral resistance which tends to restore the pressure. The heart is stimulated to increase its rate and stroke volume in an attempt to normalise output. Finally, the veins constrict, raising the venous pressure and improving ventricular filling. If the blood loss is less than one litre, these three adjustments suffice to restore normal blood pressure with a slight reduction in blood flow to most tissues.

If the loss of blood is two litres or more, the drop in cardiac output and blood pressure are substantial. Arterial constriction is unable to restore normal pressure. Cardiac stimulation increases heart rate, but with less blood returning to the heart, the stroke volume remains low however vigorous the heart muscle's contraction. Venous constriction improves ventricular filling. However, the degree of constriction needed to compensate for this blood loss begins to increase the resistance to blood flow in the veins substantially, and ventricular filling cannot be restored to normal.

In the end, the blood pressure remains sub-normal and the subject may be unable to stand without fainting. Due to low blood flow, the skin is pale and cold. The blood flow to other organs is reduced too. The pulse is hard to detect at the wrist and groin because the blood flow to the limbs is so reduced. Even the carotid pulse in the neck may be weak due to the drop in arterial pressure. Since the body's attempts to restore stroke volume are not successful, the vigorous stimulation of heart rate results in a fast pulse. In the short term the patient may appear to stabilise and even recover.

In the longer term, tissues whose blood supplies have been severely cut stage a "revolt". Their metabolic wastes accumulate and an oxygen deficit develops. In due course the vascular smooth muscle of various tissues is simply "poisoned" and relaxes, despite the vigorous stimulation from the brain telling it to constrict. When this escape from central control occurs, blood pressure drops. Because the heart can no longer compensate by increasing output, the brain blood flow falls and consciousness fades. This is called circulatory shock. If brain damage is to be avoided and survival assured, a blood transfusion is required to restore the circulating volume. In an emergency, a transfusion of saline (salt solution) may be given, but its effects last less than an hour.

Part 2 — The cardiovascular system in exercise

The cardiovascular system is responsible for a key part of the response to exercise. As oxygen consumption rises, it is the cardiovascular system's task to increase the rate at which it is brought from the lungs to the working muscles, and to return the larger quantities of waste carbon dioxide which are produced to the lungs. In addition, the supply of nutrients to fuel metabolism, such as fatty acids and glucose, must be increased. Other waste products such as potassium and heat must also be removed more rapidly, since their accumulation would hamper the high rates of metabolism required during exercise.

The supply problem in exercise is solved in two ways: the heart increases its output so that more blood is made available to carry these substances around the body, and the transport of some materials in blood is made more efficient.

Cardiac output

The cardiac output is the product of the volume pumped per stroke (stroke volume), and the number of strokes per minute (heart rate) as shown in Table 6.1.

Table 6.1

	Heart rate × stroke volume = cardiac output		
State	*(/min)*	*(ml)*	*(l/min)*
Rest	72	70	5
Moderate work	130	80	10
Maximum work	180	140	25

heart rate

At rest the heart rate is slowed by inhibitory nerve signals to around seventy beats per minute. If not for this slowing, the heart rate's "natural rythm" would be around 120/min. During physical activity this braking is released, allowing the heart to accelerate. If still higher rates are required, stimulatory nerve signals release noradrenalin at the pacemaker to speed it further. The heart rate can more than double to a maximum of between 170 and 210 beats per minute.

Table 6.2

Heart rate *(/min)*	Cycle duration *(secs)*	Duration of systole *(secs)*	*(% of cycle)*	Duration of diastole *(secs)*	*(% of cycle)*
60	1.00	0.40	40	0.60	60
120	0.50	0.28	56	0.22	44
180	0.33	0.23	70	0.10	30

As the heart rate increases, the cardiac cycle shortens (Table 6.2). However, the duration of systole is largely spared while diastole is sharply cut. Although diastole is thought of as the heart's "rest period", it is really the time available for the ventricles to fill in preparation for their next contraction.* At very high heart rates, ventricular filling becomes inefficient and the stroke volume begins to diminish. As heart rate rises above a set value (characteristic of the individual) the cardiac output fails to increase further. Heart rates over 180 beats per minute usually do

---

* Blood flows through the coronary arteries only during diastole because during systole contraction of the heart muscle squeezes them closed.

not improve pumping performance in adults, although in young children the useful maximum may exceed 220 beats per minute.

At high heart rates the atria make a useful contribution to the performance of the heart. In patients with heart block stimulatory signals from the atria fail to reach the ventricles (see p. 109). People with heart block are treated by the surgical implantation of artificial pacemakers. Some only controlled the ventricular rate, leaving atrial systole independent of the pacemaker rhythm. At rest, the long duration of diastole ensures that the atria contribute little to ventricular filling. But at high heart rates the absence of atrial assistance reduces the stroke volume by 30%. Modern pacemakers trigger from the atrial signal and synchronise atrial and ventricular systole as in the normal heart, markedly improving performance.

stroke volume
The amount of blood pumped at each heart beat can be varied. Normally, a relaxed ventricle contains about 150 ml of blood, equivalent to a full wine glass. At rest, one heart beat empties half of this, around 70 ml, into the artery. To increase stroke volume,

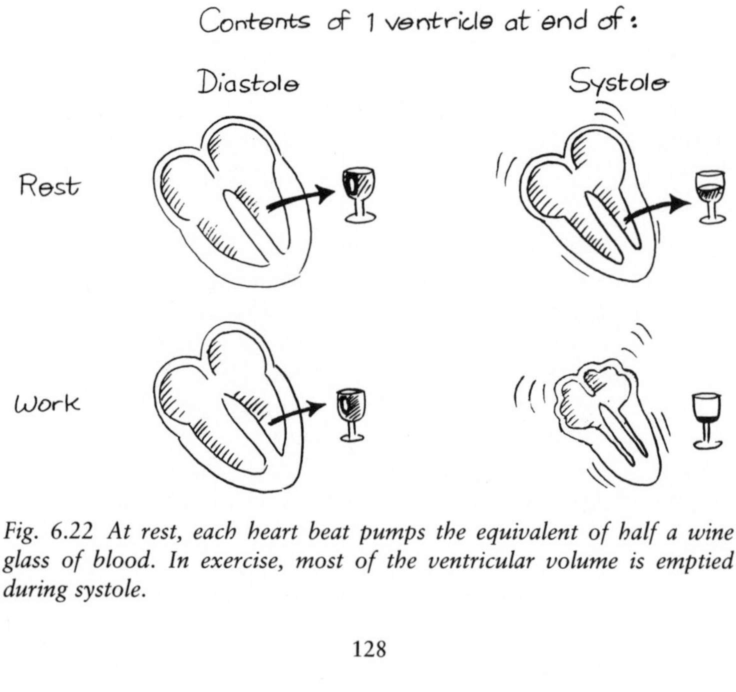

Contents of 1 ventricle at end of:

Fig. 6.22 At rest, each heart beat pumps the equivalent of half a wine glass of blood. In exercise, most of the ventricular volume is emptied during systole.

the strength of contraction must increase to allow more rapid and complete emptying, despite the reduced duration of systole (Table 6.2). At the same time, venous pressure rises (see below) to permit more rapid filling of the heart.

Increased venous pressure would stretch the ventricles and increase their volume, but for the pericardium. This inelastic membrane closely envelops the heart keeping it from stretching despite increased venous pressure. The size of the ventricles does not increase during exercise. However, following months of endurance training, the persistent stretch experienced causes the pericardium to grow, and allows the heart to enlarge or hypertrophy (see p. 140). Heart failure has a similar effect, although this is usually confined to a single ventricle.

In exercise, speeding and strengthening of the heart beat is accomplished by release into the blood of the hormone adrenalin from the adrenal gland, and of noradrenalin from stimulatory nerves ending in the heart. These hormones allow more calcium to enter the heart muscle cells, which increases the tension they can develop (see pp. 15–16). During hard work, stroke volume may double to 140 ml. Coupled with a rate of 180/min, this gives a maximum pumping performance of 25 litres (5.5 gallons) of blood per minute — for each ventricle — fast enough to fill a car's fuel tank in two to three minutes.

blood pressure
During exercise, although stroke volume increases, the volume of the large arteries doesn't change. Clearly, pushing a greater volume of blood into these vessels imposes more stretch and increases the

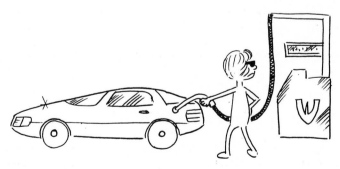

Fig. 6.23

pressure inside them. For this reason, systolic pressure rises markedly during exercise. This rise is used as a rough index of the increase in stroke volume.

Normally, the cardiac output does not increase unless and until there is a demand for additional blood flow. This demand comes from tissues with a high metabolic rate. It takes the form of an oxygen deficit and an increase in the local concentration of metabolic wastes. These cause the small arteries and arterioles within the tissue to dilate, reducing their resistance to flow so that blood flows through them in preference to other tissues whose resistance is unchanged.

In exercise, the blood vessels in working muscle are dilated and the average resistance to flow of the circulation decreases. Think of the blood flow through the body's tissues as a leak from the large arteries, and the diastolic pressure becomes an index of the size of this leak. If exercise involves a large mass of muscle, the average flow resistance of the circulation decreases sharply. This causes only a modest drop in diastolic pressure because systolic pressure rises, and the duration of diastole is shortened at the same time.

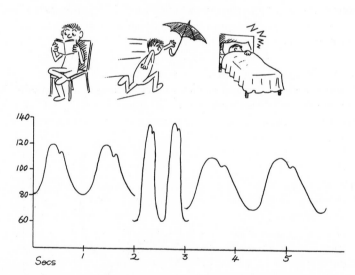

Fig. 6.24 In exercise the systolic pressure rises and the diastolic pressure falls. By contrast, during sleep, when the metabolic rate and the cardiac output are low, both pressures fall.

venous return mirrors cardiac output

Everybody is aware of the increased heart rate which accompanies exercise. Many people are also aware of the pounding pulse which is a sign of the increase in stroke volume. However, the heart cannot pump more blood than it receives, and any increase in output must be matched by a similar increase in the volume of blood returning to the heart. (It is also obvious that the volume pumped by the left and the right sides of the heart must be identical otherwise the lungs would either fill up with blood, or empty.)

The rate at which blood returns to the heart depends upon the venous blood pressure. The higher this is, the faster blood returns. As the arterioles and capillaries in working muscle dilate and fill with blood, volume is transferred from the venous reservoir, reducing its pressure. In exercise this small loss of venous volume and pressure must be made up. Then pressure must be raised further, above resting values, to cater for the increase in cardiac output.

Venous pressure is raised by several means. First is the direct effect of the skeletal muscles through which many veins run. As a muscle contracts, these veins are squeezed, and with the help of the venous valves, flow towards the heart is greatly improved and the venous pressure increases (Fig. 6.16) — an automatic result of exercise. Venous pressure is also increased by contraction of vessel smooth muscle under the influence of noradrenalin. Normally, veins are oval in cross-section and incompletely full. This gives them great scope for contraction while causing little change in flow resistance.

Finally, the rate at which blood returns to the heart depends upon the pressure inside the heart as well as on the pressure in veins. During breathing, pressure within the chest drops below atmospheric to induce air to enter the lungs. The average pressure inside the heart is influenced by respiration. During inspiration, blood flow into the thorax therefore increases, assisting right ventricular filling (Fig. 6.25), and increasing the volume of blood in the lungs. During expiration thoracic pressure rises squeezing blood out of the lung, assisting left ventricular filling. Thus, respiratory movements aid the filling of both ventricles. During exercise, respiratory movements become both frequent and powerful, and the thoracic pumping action becomes more effective.

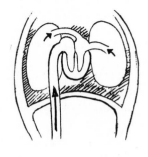

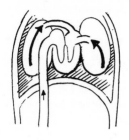

Inspiration   Expiration

Fig. 6.25 The thoracic pressure rises and falls during breathing. At inspiration thoracic pressure falls, drawing venous blood into the chest and filling the lungs. At expiration it rises, pushing blood from the lungs into the left ventricle.

A final factor is related to the heat generated during exercise. This is partly dissipated by evaporation of sweat from the skin. The resulting fluid loss can lead to a considerable reduction in plasma volume, making it difficult for the heart to maintain a high cardiac output (see Ch. 8).

where does the cardiac output go?
The cardiac output is the amount of blood pumped each minute by each ventricle of the heart. The output of the left ventricle is distributed to the various organs of the body according to their needs. In general, the greater the metabolic rate of a tissue, the greater its requirement for oxygen and blood flow. (Of course, the output of the right ventricle is exactly equal to that of the left, and flows through the lungs.)

Certain tissues use their blood flow for purposes other than the supply of oxygen and nutrients. Thus, at rest, the kidney receives 22% of the cardiac output but is responsible for just 7% of the resting oxygen consumption. Most of the kidney's blood flow is provided for the purpose of "cleansing" the blood. In exercise this job is curtailed and may even be abandoned so that much of the kidney's blood flow can be diverted to muscle.

The skin loses heat to the environment at a rate proportional to

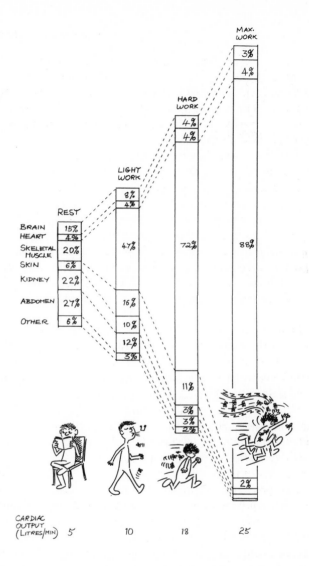

Fig. 6.26 *Cardiac output increases with the vigour of exercise, and an estimate of its value is given at the bottom of the figure. The distribution of blood flow in the body also changes. Estimates of the percentage of total flow going to each region are given. Note that: (1) brain blood flow remains constant; (2) supply to the heart is proportional to the heart's work; (3) blood flow through "less important" tissues (kidney, abdomen, etc.) decreases; (4) skin flow increases to dissipate the heat produced, except during maximum work (which anyway cannot be sustained).*

its blood flow. The oxygen requirement of skin is small and barely rises with activity, but its blood flow during exercise is more than eight times greater than at rest. In maximal work the skin blood flow and thermoregulation are forsaken (Fig. 6.26) because this rate of work cannot be sustained for long. In emergencies, the body simply allows itself to heat up for a limited time (Ch. 7).

At rest, it is clear that most organs and tissues receive a blood flow closely related to their metabolic needs (Fig. 6.26). During exercise, tissues not directly involved in the effort (gut, liver, kidney) are deprived of much of their blood supply as a result of general vascular constriction. The brain is not deprived of blood flow, and has a delightfully simple technique to guarantee its supply. If the demand for blood flow outstrips the cardiac output — that is, if the output is too low to maintain blood pressure — fainting occurs and the head drops. This increases pressure at the cerebral arteries and tends to maintain the cerebral flow!

Control of the exercising cardiovascular system

The cardiovascular system receives two sorts of pressure information. Arterial baroreceptors in the aorta and carotid arteries detect the pressure of the blood immediately after the heart. Meanwhile, venous and atrial receptors measure the degree of stretch within the large veins and the heart's atria and treat this as a representation of the volume of the venous system.

However, cardiovascular performance is not gauged by internal pressures, but by the adequacy of blood flow delivered to its client tissues. The body has no means of sensing blood flow directly but, during exercise, the increased metabolic rate uses more oxygen and produces more waste products. The resting blood flow becomes inadequate to support the requirements of active tissues. The consequence is a lack of oxygen and a rising concentration of metabolic waste products within working muscle (p. 122). These local environmental changes cause the small arteries serving the tissue to dilate, reducing resistance and bringing more blood flow. The blood flow continues to increase until the local environment achieves a more satisfactory concentration of oxygen and wastes.

Muscle forms a large proportion of the body's mass. Reduction of flow resistance simultaneously in many muscles could cause a dangerous drop in blood pressure. Baroreceptors detect this as it develops and warn the brain to:

1. stimulate the heart to contract more frequently and more vigorously, increasing cardiac output,
2. constrict other blood vessels, diverting more cardiac output to the working muscles, and,
3. constrict the veins to improve venous pressure and the filling of the heart.

These responses can cause the cardiac output to increase by up to five-fold, and prevent any drop in the blood pressure.

cardiovascular efficiency in exercise and its importance
When the demand for blood flow from a particular region is high, the overall level of vasoconstrictor signals from the brain is also

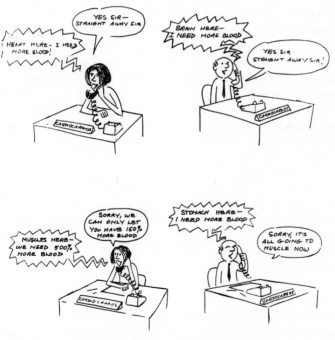

Fig. 6.27 *The brain and the heart apart, the blood supplies of most other tissues are either reduced, or are less than they "desire".*

high. Organs which are at rest therefore experience a decrease in blood supply. This, in turn, increases the local concentration of metabolic wastes. The degree to which the blood flow in a tissue may be reduced is limited by the oxygen depletion and waste accumulation which it can tolerate.

The working muscles whose heavy demand originated the re-adjustment in cardiovascular performance also receive a barrage of vasoconstrictor signals. Consequently, although their blood flow is high, it is less than they "demand". In other words, despite the increased blood flow in working muscle, the local concentration of metabolites during exercise rises compared to rest.

This condition of deprivation is important. By restricting the rate of blood flow to working muscles and other tissues with high rates of metabolism, the cardiovascular system forces them to extract more oxygen from their blood supply. Since the overall metabolic rate in exercise can rise sixteen-fold while the perform-ance of the cardiovascular system is limited to a five-fold increase, an improvement in oxygen extraction is vital (see Ch. 5), and is the means by which the body makes efficient use of the limited cardiac output available to it.

At rest, the kidneys, weighing less than one pound, receive over one litre of blood flow per minute, or 25% of the cardiac output. This lavish blood supply is used to filter the blood and to form urine. During exercise kidney blood flow is cut to a quarter of the resting value, just enough to supply the tissue with oxygen. The kidney abandons its normal work in exercise, liberating most of its share of the cardiac output for the use of muscle.

The brain's central control wages a constant "battle" with the demands of the local control systems. If uncontrolled, local blood flow would be high enough to keep the concentration of wastes at a needlessly low level. This would impose unrealistic, and often unattainable output demands on the heart. This is similar to the conflict between central and local government where the latter might have a long list of electorally desirable projects which the former must trim according to the available resources.

In summary, the best possible cardiovascular performance is not enough to cope with maximum demands from all of the tissues. The central control system solves this problem by meeting none of these demands in full apart from those of the brain and heart.

velocity of blood flow during exercise

It is worth noting that increasing the rate of blood flow through a tissue often doesn't increase the velocity of flow in the small blood vessels (Fig. 6.28). High speed flow would reduce the efficiency of diffusion. Instead, flow is increased by opening up more arterioles and their capillary beds so that more capillaries carry the flow than before. This also means that cells in the tissue find themselves closer to a supply of fresh blood, reducing the diffusion distance and speeding the exchange of materials (pp. 82, 139).

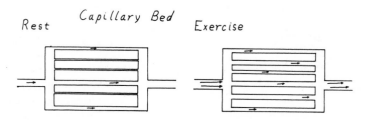

Fig. 6.28 An increased rate of blood flow doesn't mean higher flow velocity.

Effects of training on the cardiovascular system

strength training

The main cardiovascular effect of strength training is on the heart itself. The classic form of strength training is weight lifting in which brief intervals of intense activity are separated by relatively long periods of rest. A high rate of oxygen consumption is never achieved, providing little stimulus for training the cardiovascular system.

During a heavy lift many of the body's muscles are powerfully contracted, squeezing the arteries passing through them, and greatly increasing vascular resistance. Accordingly, the blood pressure rises steeply, making it harder for the heart to discharge its stroke volume. In response to these repeated episodes of high blood pressure the heart muscle enlarges and strengthens by hypertrophy. This means that individual muscle fibres become thicker and stronger. The volume of wrestlers and weight lifters' ventricles are similar to (or even smaller than) those of sedentary people. However, the total weight of their cardiac muscle is considerably greater, particularly in the left ventricle.

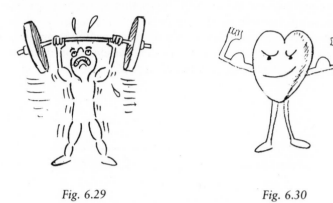

Fig. 6.29   Fig. 6.30

The larger heart muscle fibres characteristic of strength trained athletes can be at a metabolic disadvantage. Their increased thickness means that the centres of these muscle cells are farther from their capillaries (see p. 18). Oxygen takes longer to diffuse in, and waste products to diffuse out, limiting their metabolic performance. It has even been suggested that this poor diffusion may put strength athletes at increased risk of coronary heart disease, but evidence for this is inconclusive.

endurance training
Whether you are an office worker, boilermaker, postman, or school athlete, training can improve your cardiovascular performance. Endurance training affects the whole cardiovascular system: volume, capillaries, heart and control system.
(a) plasma volume
     Within ten days of starting endurance training, the plasma volume increases by 10–15% while the number of red blood cells increases by less. For this reason, endurance athletes tend to have slightly reduced concentrations of haemoglobin. In effect this is a mild anaemia, giving endurance athletes a lower blood viscosity than the population average.
     Some people believe that the mild apparent anaemia of

138

athletes is caused by the loss of haemoglobin in the stool and urine. They suggest that the lost haemoglobin comes from red cells damaged in a runner's pounding feet, or from organs which were hypoxic during exercise as a result of the diversion of blood flow from them to working muscle. Athletes probably do lose some haemoglobin in this way, but the amounts involved are very small. Their mild anaemia is due simply to the increase in plasma volume exceeding that of the red cells, and may be an adaptation which improves endurance.

The maintenance of a high cardiac output depends on the efficient return of venous blood to the heart. As water is lost from the body in sweat, the concentration of red cells in the blood increases, making the blood more viscous (see p. 181). Simultaneously, the loss of blood volume reduces venous pressure. Together, these two changes reduce the rate at which blood returns to the heart. Trained endurance athletes, who start out with reduced blood viscosity and increased plasma volume, can continue to pump a high cardiac output for a longer period of time when a large volume of sweat is being produced.

(b) capillary density

Endurance training increases the density of capillaries in exercised muscle (Fig. 6.31). During work the concentration of oxygen in muscle is reduced. Periodic hypoxia in training stimulates capillaries to grow through the muscle, bringing the blood supply closer to individual muscle cells. (Capillary growth also occurs in patients with heart disease whose cardiac output is reduced through illness, and in natives of high altitude environments where the oxygen supply is poor.) This effect is largely confined to the slow muscle fibres which respond best to endurance training. The blood supply of fast

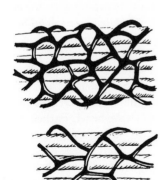

Fig. 6.31 Endurance trained muscles develop additional capillaries, reducing the diffusion distance for nutrients and respiratory gases.

139

"sprint" muscle fibres is little changed by endurance training.

During exercise blood flow through muscle increases. If this simply raised the velocity of flow in capillaries, then the time available for diffusion would be reduced, making the exchange of materials inefficient. The greater number of capillaries available ensures that when the muscle's demand for blood flow is increased, this flow will find additional channels to take and not simply speed (ineffectually) through the muscle (Fig. 6.28).

The main result of the increase in capillary density is a marked reduction in the diffusion distance between capillary and muscle cell. This allows smaller differences in concentration to drive the movement of materials. One effect is that endurance trained muscles can remove more oxygen from their blood supply than can those of sedentary people. Similarly, the muscles of endurance athletes can continue to get rid of lactic acid when its concentration in the blood has become high enough to disable metabolism in a sedentary individual.

This last consequence of endurance training — increased capillary density — may be even more important to an athlete than any improvement in the performance of the heart.

(c) heart muscle

As with any muscle, exercising the heart strengthens it. What actually happens is that hard work causes the cells in heart muscle to produce more contractile protein and to grow thicker. This is called hypertrophy. When hypertrophied hearts are stimulated to contract, they can develop more tension than untrained heart muscle. This means that they are capable of emptying more rapidly and more completely during the course of systole.

In exercise, the pressure within the veins increases to encourage more rapid return of blood to the heart. Earlier it was stated (p. 129) that the pericardium prevents the heart from stretching. However, subjecting the heart to a persistently raised filling pressure causes the pericardium to grow and allows the ventricles to increase their volume. This increase in ventricular volume and the simultaneous development of enough strength to pump it increases the stroke volume. Hence, the resting cardiac output of five litres per minute is produced at a lower heart rate. A low resting heart rate is characteristic of physically fit individuals. Resting rates in the

50s or lower are common among athletes, implying resting stroke volumes of over 100 ml, instead of the usual 70 ml.

Individuals with hearts capable of large stroke volumes can obviously produce large cardiac outputs and support high rates of work. What is just as important is that such people can deliver high cardiac outputs without having to resort to very fast heart rates which are themselves disadvantageous (Table 6.2).

Excessive endurance training can lead to the development of "athletes heart". Athletes with this condition have: a very slow heart rate (less than 40/min); hypertrophy of the heart muscle; and partial heart block. A group of sixteen athletes who suffered from fainting spells all had resting heart rates lower than 40 beats/min and suffered from partial heart block (p. 108). Seven of them had pacemakers implanted for this life-threatening condition, while the rest recovered after moderating their training. A subsequent survey of a larger group of athletes, 25% of whom had heart rates lower than 40/min, showed that 20% had "ventricular pauses" (periods between beats) longer than two seconds, and were thought to be at risk of developing heart block.

The very low heart rates characteristic of athletes may lead to dangerous rhythm problems. This vividly illustrates that anything, however beneficial, can be overdone.

(d) blood pressure

Blood pressure rises during activity. Systolic pressure rises substantially, while diastolic pressure remains unchanged or may even diminish slightly. During activity the systolic pressure of mild hypertensives rises to the same final value as that of exercising normotensives. So there is no reason for mildly hypertensive individuals to abstain from exercise for fear of the consequences of high blood pressure.

In America, life insurance policies are popular and the premiums are based on the results of regular medical examinations. People with high blood pressure pay high premiums. Some years ago it was observed that, following an hour's jogging, the blood pressure drops to below pre-exercise values, and remains low for several hours. This enabled the mildly hypertensive individual to schedule a run before his/her doctor's appointment, saving on the annual insurance premium!

Regular endurance training reduces resting blood pressure. This effect may be quite large in people with higher blood pressures, although a small response occurs in all people. It has been reported that in moderate hypertensives who undertake daily exercise, the effect may be large enough to allow a reduction in the dose of antihypertensive medication.

It is difficult to assign responsibility for the decrease in blood pressure. Whether this is due directly to changes in cardiovascular performance or to changes in diet, smoking, sleep habits, weight, anxiety, etc., associated with the training regime, is not known. Considering the cost of lifelong antihypertensive medication and its side effects, exercise is certainly worth trying in selected patients, whatever the mechanism behind the improvement.

Is training worthwhile?

what is achieved?

Training achieves only relatively small improvements in cardiovascular performance: 10% greater cardiac output, an extra half-litre of plasma, some additional capillaries in muscle. Is it worthwhile? Well, these effects add together and give the sedentary individual who completes a training regime a clear and marked improvement in both speed and endurance.

One recent study persuaded thirty-nine sedentary (no regular exercise for at least two years) and middle-aged (average age 40) men to train under supervision for thirty weeks. Initially, they were only able to manage three twenty-minute runs each week, and we can imagine that each run left them pretty tired! After twenty weeks, they were running faster, six times a week, and for an hour at a time.

In another study undertaken at an Australian military camp, fifty young men (average age 21) were given two weeks of training requiring three circuits of a ten station course to be performed twice daily. Each station consisted of a physical task such as "chin-ups", "press-ups", etc. Immediately after a session, pulse rates were around 170 beats per minute. Physical fitness was gauged by the rate at which the pulse rate recovered.

At the start of training, the pulse rate of the new trainees

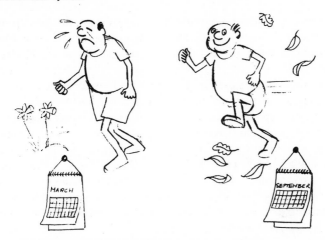

Fig. 6.32 *Developing physical fitness can take as little as two to three weeks, although several months may be required, depending on the starting point and standard of fitness desired. Usually, there is no weight loss (see Ch. 10).*

remained over 100/min even after ten minutes of rest. Within two weeks, the pulse rate measured after ten minutes of rest dropped to 80/min. Using a fitness index based on pulse rates at 2, 5, and 10 minutes, a mere six hours of training spread over two weeks gave a 20% improvement in fitness. Performance also improved. At the start of the programme each circuit took twelve minutes. By one week each circuit took 8.5 minutes; and after two weeks, under eight minutes. Based on these circuit times, this brief period of training gave the subjects a 30% improvement in speed as well as a faster rate of recovery!

the collective effect is the sum of its parts

Clearly, the cardiovascular system responds to training, but the individual changes which may be measured are small. However, overall track performance is often substantially improved. Training also changes metabolic performance, and the characteristics of skeletal muscle.

Consider the twin changes of increased cardiac output and increased capillary density. Increased capillary density enables working muscle to extract more oxygen from the same rate of

143

blood flow — perhaps an extra 10%. In addition, the heart is able to pump 10% more blood, all of which is available to working muscle. The total effect gives the working muscles 20% more oxygen.

Even this explains only part of the improvement in performance. It is impossible to train the cardiovascular system without also training the rest of the body. Thus, metabolic changes (see Ch. 3) allow muscle to take energy from fat rather than carbohydrate, and to improve aerobic capacity (ability to use oxygen), so that work causes less lactic acid to be produced. Both of these metabolic adaptations improve endurance. Skeletal muscle hypertrophies increasing strength and reducing fatigue. Skill also improves, making the individual more efficient at the specific activity so that less energy is required. Consequently, it is hard to separate the contribution to performance of the trained cardiovascular system from the contributions of other systems.

Genetics and the cardiovascular system

In ordinary mortals the maximum cardiac output is 20–25 litres per minute for a 70 kg male, and 14–18 litres per minute for a 60 kg female. Measurements on international endurance athletes have found cardiac outputs of 30–45 litres per minute in males and 20–30 litres per minute in females.

No amount of training will develop the cardiac output of an ordinary person, however determined, up to those seen in competitive athletes. Typically, training gives a 10% increase in cardiac output, although this is accompanied by a far greater improvement in track performance. The cardiovascular development which can be achieved depends on the original level of fitness. Although the sedentary have scope for greater improvement than more active people, they often lack the necessary determination. The exceptional cardiovascular performance of competitive endurance athletes is partly the product of intensive training, but is mainly due to their superior genetic inheritance.

The majority of endurance athletes are not aware of their high powered cardiovascular systems because the required measurements are seldom made. In school, they probably performed unexceptionally in discus throwing and jumping, but showed special aptitude for endurance events. If they chose to continue in competition, this would most likely be in those activities where their cardiac output (unknown to themselves) gave them some special advantage.

In the population there must be many people with exceptional cardiovascular systems who had neither the opportunity nor the inclination to compete in endurance sport. Their cardiovascular capabilities (and athletic potential) remain undiscovered. However, a few sedentary siblings of champion endurance athletes have been investigated in the laboratory and were found to have cardiac outputs well above the population average — and wasted on people with no interest in sport!

One reason why relatively small countries like East Germany and Cuba have done so well in international athletics is that they patiently search their school children for individuals with both exceptional ability and physiological capacity. These are then given the opportunity to train and compete. Such countries also reward their athletes in various ways, further encouraging them to take up the sports opportunities on offer.

Summary

The cardiovascular system is usually the limiting factor in aerobic work. Initially, aerobic work is limited by the supply of oxygen rather than the ability to use oxygen. Endurance training enlarges the heart, increasing its output, and allowing the maximum output to be achieved at lower heart rates. Meanwhile, more capillaries grow into the trained muscle. Their high density allows materials to be exchanged more efficiently, so that less blood flow is required to support any rate of activity. Together, these changes increase the maximum rate of aerobic work which the cardiovascular system can support. Coupled with changes in skill (hence work efficiency) and muscle strength, performance (capacity to do work) must improve.

In endurance work, the continuous loss of water as sweat increases blood viscosity, reduces volume and gradually lowers the output of the heart. Eventually work rate and the ability to cool the body suffer, marking the limit of endurance. The high blood volume and slight anaemia characteristic of trained athletes delays this limit, prolonging performance. Endurance is also the product of metabolic change favouring the use of fat as a fuel and of reducing the amount of lactic acid accumulated during work.

Although an improvement in cardiovascular performance is attainable through endurance training, it is not normally possible for an individual to achieve the level of cardiovascular performance characteristic of competitive athletes. Champion endurance athletes probably inherit their exceptional cardiovascular systems, and training simply serves to hone them to peak performance.

CHAPTER SEVEN

Temperature regulation

Background

When a cell cools, its chemical reactions slow markedly. For hundreds of millions of years animals warmed themselves cheaply using the heat of the sun. During this long period of time a variety of thermoregulatory techniques evolved to speed warming and to enable animals to become active earlier in the day. All of these were, however, dependent on free solar energy.

In the cool temperature of early morning, "cold-blooded" animals such as lizards, frogs, and tortoises may be seen moving sluggishly, searching for a warm, sunny spot in which to bask. For these animals basking is not leisure, but an important prelude to the foraging day. Animals which remain cold and in a state of torpor will become breakfast for their warm, alert neighbours.

The first mammals and birds represented a biological revolution in which the regulation of body temperature became an active process where heat was generated within the body by a high rate

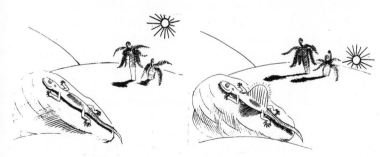

Fig. 7.1 Early schemes for thermo-regulation were accomplished by basking in the sun until the correct body temperature was achieved.

Fig. 7.2 One improved basking scheme used a vertical "sail" to catch the light. This allowed the animal to warm up sooner, and perhaps eat his less advanced neighbour.

F

of metabolism (10–20 times that of comparable reptiles), and retained by efficient insulation (feathers, fur, or fat). This meant that a stable temperature could be maintained day and night, regardless of climate or season. "Warm-blooded" animals were able to forage and hunt under conditions in which the "cold-blooded" competition was helpless.*

Once evolution had devised mechanisms for maintaining a high metabolic rate, these were hard to turn off. Mammalian metabolic chemistry, adapted to a constant and high body temperature, was less able to tolerate a fall in temperature (or a rise) than was the old reptilian metabolism. Thus, few mammals are able to slow metabolism when their temperature is high. In parallel with the trend to high metabolic rates, efficient and reliable cooling systems had to evolve.

Thermoregulation in mammals is a complex response combining control of metabolic heat generation, with the ability to distribute heat around the body and very effective methods of heat dissipation.

How much heat do we produce?

The energy for movement, tissue repair, growth and supporting activities (eg. cardiovascular, digestive and respiratory work, transport of materials across cells, etc.) all comes from food. By means of chemical reactions catalysed by enzymes (Ch. 3), food is "burned" at low temperature converting fats, carbohydrates, and proteins into water, carbon dioxide, and energy (including heat).

The energy intake can be easily and accurately determined by weighing the food eaten. In fully grown adults, with the exception of small losses (hair, fingernails, skin) and some digestive inefficiency, this energy duly appears either as heat or as external work (movement). On average, physical activity is around 15% efficient, leaving 85% of the energy to be dissipated as heat. Even so, physical activity usually accounts for less (often markedly less) than one third of the total energy expenditure (Ch. 3). So the

---

* It is now believed that dinosaurs were "warm-blooded", and capable of maintaining high rates of metabolism. If true, this might partly explain why they were able to dominate the world for 130 million years.

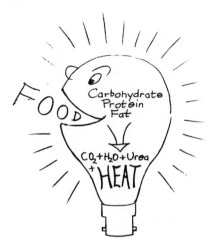

$\male$ 2400 kcal/day of heat is equivalent to 115 Watts

$\female$ 1800 kcal/day of heat is equivalent to 85 Watts

Fig. 7.3 Our resting heat production is approximately the same as that of a light bulb.

assumption that energy intake is equal to heat production involves little error:

ENERGY INTAKE = HEAT OUTPUT

In females, the daily intake of food amounts to 1800 kilocalories per day (kcal/day); in males, this is 2400 kcal/day. On the other hand, heat production is generally expressed in Watts, a unit with which most people are familiar. Since one Watt is one Joule per second, and 4.186 Joules = 1 Calorie, energy intakes can be converted into Watts. The average rate of heat production over a 24-hour day is 85 Watts for women and 115 Watts for men.

For a small object such as a light bulb this rate of heat production is high, and its surface must become quite hot to dissipate the heat. However, for a human body with a relatively large surface area, this rate of heat production is low, and even in warm

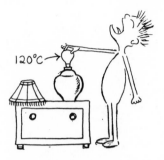

120°C →

Fig. 7.4 For a person with a surface area of 1.5–2.0 square metres, 100 Watts is a low rate of heat production and our skin temperature might be 25°C. On the other hand, a 100 Watt light bulb must dissipate the same amount of heat over a very small surface, and its temperature exceeds 100°C.

environments we require some insulation in order to remain comfortable. In winter a lot of clothing must be worn to maintain our body temperature at its normal value with this modest metabolic rate.

Heat production is variable. The metabolic rate is particularly low at night. This is referred to as the Basal Metabolic Rate or BMR. The BMR is around 50 Watts for women and 65 Watts for men. During activity this can rise dramatically. Maximum values for normal individuals (non-athletes) are 1000 Watts in women, and 1300 Watts in men, or twenty times the BMR. Such rates of activity cannot be sustained for long, partly because of fatigue and partly due to the problem of dissipating the large amount of heat produced.

The physics of heat dissipation

Heat is transferred from one body to another in several ways: by conduction, convection, and by radiation. These operate wherever a temperature difference or gradient exists. Heat can also be lost by evaporation.

conduction and convection

Heat flows or is conducted from a warm object to a cool one. The rate of heat transfer depends on the temperature difference between the

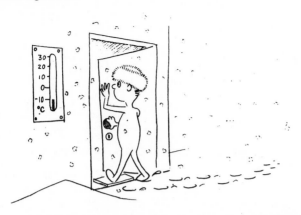

Fig. 7.5 CONDUCTION: *high conductivity makes a brass doorknob feel far colder than a low conductivity wooden door, although both actually have the same temperature.*

objects, their thermal conductivity, and the area over which they contact each other.

Convection is similar to conduction. Heat is transferred between a body and the fluid in which it is immersed. Since the fluid moves, fresh material is constantly brought into contact with the body. Thus, on a windy day, it always feels far colder than the temperature would suggest.

radiation

Radiation can transfer heat between two objects which are not in contact. The amount of heat transferred depends on the 4th power of the temperature difference between the objects. Clearly, this becomes very much more effective as the temperature gradient increases. For example, if the temperature of a heater in a 20°C room increases from 220°C to 420°C, its heat loss by convection and conduction doubles, while its radiation increases sixteen times!

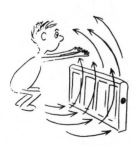

Fig. 7.6 CONVECTION: *heated by the radiator, air rises and is replaced by a fresh supply of cool air. The warm air may then transfer heat to another body by convection.*

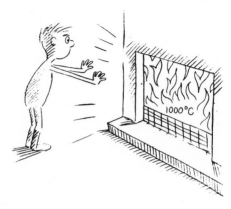

Fig. 7.7 RADIATION: in the absence of physical contact, heat is transferred by radiation.

Most animals, including man, are poorly equipped to lose heat by radiation. However, we do take advantage of solar radiation when basking on a sunny beach. On a sunny day, radiant heat gain may add considerably to an athlete's cooling burden.

evaporation

Evaporation transfers heat by converting water from a liquid into its vapour state. This takes approximately 550 kcal or 2300 Joules for each litre of water evaporated (depending on the temperature at which this is done). Vapourizing one litre of water requires the heat equivalent to 25% of one day's energy intake. This is a powerful method of heat loss, used when other methods cannot cope. It is limited only by the quantity of water the body can afford to lose (Ch. 8). Evaporation is required at high temperatures when sufficient heat cannot be lost to the environment by conduction. Indeed, heat cannot be lost by conduction or convection at all when the environmental temperature rises much over 30°C (Fig. 7.11).

The body uses all of these methods of heat loss to some extent. Normally, most of our heat loss is by convection to air — the layer of warm air trapped by our clothing next to the body. In summer, to improve heat loss we cover less of our bodies, and wear better ventilated clothing. In windy weather, the warm air trapped by our clothing is stirred by movement, and partly replaced by cool air, reducing the insulating quality of a garment.

152

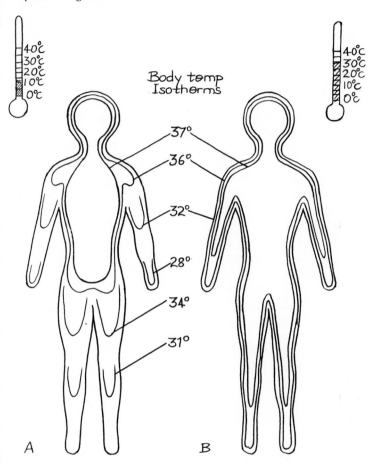

Fig. 7.8 Temperature "Isotherms" (lines of equal temperature) in the body. In a cool environment, the warm core of the body retreats and the skin and the limbs are far cooler than on a warm day.

How do we regulate temperature?

what is body temperature?

We are said to have a constant and well regulated body temperature, to the point where temperature is used as a reliable indicator of illness. In fact, the body temperature is not as steady as the arrow on a clinical thermometer might lead one to believe. It falls from around 37°C during the day to 36°C at night. In women a sharp 0.3°C rise in temperature can be used to detect the time of ovulation. During hard work, the body's temperature can rise by as much as 3°C.

Various parts of the body are kept at different temperatures. The oral or rectal temperature commonly measured (supposedly the temperature of arterial blood or "core" temperature) is lower than that of tissues with high metabolic rates which generate a great deal of heat. Skin, particularly where it is exposed to a cold environment is far cooler than the core temperature. Limbs also tend to be cooler than the core (Fig. 7.8). However, during work, when they are generating heat, working muscles become very warm and may exceed 40°C.

heat loss from the body, an overview
Heat dissipation from the body proceeds in two stages, and is similar to cooling a car engine. In the car, heat from combustion is first transferred to the water jacket surrounding the cylinders. This water is then circulated through the radiator. Engine temperature is kept constant by a thermostat which regulates water flow through the radiator. A second thermostat monitors the temperature of the radiator. When this becomes too warm, an electric fan is turned on to cool the radiator.

In the body, the first stage of heat dissipation transfers metabolic heat to the skin by the flow of blood. The blood flow to each tissue is controlled by metabolic demand, and any shortfall in blood flow would limit the metabolic rate (Ch. 5). For this reason,

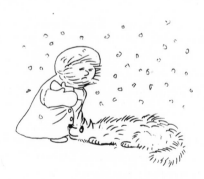

Fig. 7.9

the rate of blood flow through a tissue is automatically adequate for cooling.

The second stage of heat dissipation controls skin temperature, ensuring that the difference in temperature between the skin and the blood flowing through it is large enough to cool the blood, and the body. The temperature gradient between the skin and the arterial blood varies, but it is usually at least 4°C. The minimum rate of blood flow to the skin is about 300 ml/min or 18 l/hr. This gives an average rate of heat delivery to the skin of about $4 \times 18 = 72$ kcal/hr*, and must closely match the average resting metabolic rate (estimated as 75 kcal/hr — Ch. 3).

adjusting the rate of heat loss

On entering a cold environment, the skin cools and the amount of heat being lost by the blood flowing through it increases. Since the skin blood flow cannot be reduced much below 300 ml/min., to prevent the body from cooling the skin must be insulated with clothing to raise its temperature (animals fluff up their fur). Alternatively, the countercurrent heat exchange system may be activated (see below).

In a hot environment the skin warms. Since the rate at which heat is brought to the skin depends partly on the difference in

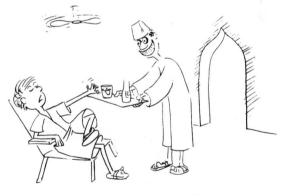

Fig. 7.10

---

* A kilocalorie (kcal) is the amount of heat required to raise the temperature of one kilogram of water by one centigrade degree.

COLD

Metabolic Heat Production	110 watts
Evaporation 13%	14 watts
Convection/Conduction 26%	29 watts
Radiation 61%	67 watts

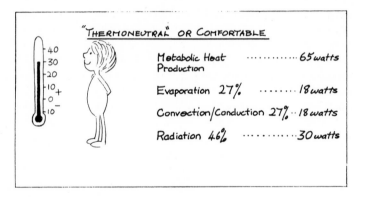

"THERMONEUTRAL" OR COMFORTABLE

Metabolic Heat Production	65 watts
Evaporation 27%	18 watts
Convection/Conduction 27%	18 watts
Radiation 46%	30 watts

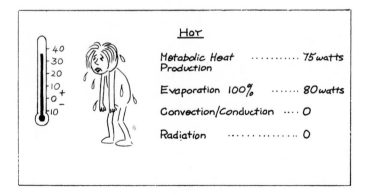

HOT

Metabolic Heat Production	75 watts
Evaporation 100%	80 watts
Convection/Conduction	0
Radiation	0

temperature between the skin and the blood, heat transfer diminishes. Increasing the flow of blood to the skin delivers more heat, but also raises skin temperature further. As skin temperature rises, the cooling of the body becomes inadequate.

To maintain cooling, skin temperature must be reduced. Clothing may be removed, convection may be improved by opening a window, or sweat may be formed to cool the skin by evaporation. Skin temperature is monitored by skin sensors which send information to a part of the brain called the hypothalamus. When the skin becomes too warm, the hypothalamus initiates sweating to cool it.

Physiology of thermoregulation in detail

Cooling is only part of temperature regulation. We must also maintain the body temperature in cool environments when our level of activity is low. Thermoregulation is controlled by a centre in the brain called the hypothalamus which measures the temperature of the brain's blood supply. The hypothalamus also receives information on skin temperatures around the body, and integrates this data to produce a thermoregulatory response. The complete spectrum of responses the body has to regulate heat production and loss are:

1. Control of skin blood flow
2. Regulation of metabolic rate

Fig. 7.11 This shows the amount of heat lost by an unclothed 70 kg male by the 3 routes (radiation, conduction and convection, evaporation), at three environmental temperatures. At 30°C, a nude subject is comfortable and the metabolic rate is at its basal (lowest) value of 65 Watts. Temperatures around 30°C are called thermoneutral. The heat loss is divided, with 46% by radiation, and 27% each for convection and evaporation (there is a minimum rate of evaporation from the skin and the respiratory system, even at cool temperatures). At 20°C, a nude subject feels cold and the metabolic rate rises in compensation to about 110 Watts. The heat loss is 61% by radiation, 26% by convection and 13% by evaporation (again minimal). At 36°C, the metabolic rate of 75 Watts is higher than the basal value because heat loss requires energy (sweating, high skin blood flow). Here 100% of the heat produced must be lost by evaporation because sweating makes the skin cooler than the environment and the subject may even gain some heat from the surroundings.

3. Countercurrent heat exchange mechanism
4. Sweat production
5. Shelter.

skin blood flow

Warm blood from the body flows through the skin, is cooled, and returns to the body to cool metabolically active tissues. In order to cool properly, the temperature of the skin must be maintained at 4–6°C below that of the arterial blood. (Note: The arterial blood flow to a limb, and the skin covering it, may be quite cool — see countercurrent heat exchange below.)

When the environment is cold and the metabolic rate is low, blood flow to the skin is minimised and controlled by its own small oxygen requirement. If skin temperature drops below freezing, permanent damage (frostbite) can occur. The Inuit (Eskimos) are resistant to this, maintaining some blood flow to the skin under cold conditions to prevent freezing — and accepting the heat loss. By contrast, negroes are susceptible to frostbite, physiologically putting a higher priority on heat conservation than on the health of the skin. In tropical Africa, the negroes rarely suffered freezing conditions and experienced no evolutionary pressure to protect against it. Caucasians (whites) lie between these extremes.

If either the environmental temperature or the metabolic rate increase, the hypothalamus detects the rising blood temperature, and increases skin blood flow, thereby increasing the delivery of heat to the skin and warming it. At this point the skin blood flow is dictated by the needs of thermoregulation, and may be well in excess of its own small metabolic requirement.

regulation of the metabolic rate

The metabolism is our personal central heating system, and the metabolic rate is the speed at which fuel is burned. When the environmental temperature falls, the metabolic rate increases to help maintain body temperature. There are several ways in which this response is brought about.

The rise in metabolic rate during exercise can maintain body temperature under quite cold conditions. For example, the skimpy clothing of football players in winter is clearly adequate because their metabolic rate is high.

Random muscle contractions which produce no real movement also increase heat production in the cold. This is shivering and although rare in today's centrally heated society, it was common enough not long ago. Shivering is also seen in feverish people where, although the body temperature is high, a reset control system perceives it as low and attempts to warm the body further.

Exposure to cold causes the release of the hormone adrenalin which makes the metabolic rate rise rapidly, but briefly. Prolonged cold exposure gradually increases the production of thyroid hormone, which also stimulates metabolism. It is not certain which chemical reactions are stimulated, but these may involve burning metabolic fuel without producing ATP — purely for heat. Thus, American soldiers stationed in Alaska during winter eat nearly twice as much as their compatriots in Florida, vividly illustrating the metabolic stimulation which a cold climate may cause.

Although metabolism is stimulated in a cold environment, the opposite does not occur in a hot climate. In fact, getting rid of heat costs the body extra work, so the metabolic rate rises slightly at high temperatures (Fig. 7.11). No matter how warm the environment, the metabolic rate cannot be reduced below its basal value in man (although high temperature does cause the metabolic rate to fall in certain African antelope). The basal metabolic rate can be reduced by starvation, but not in response to high temperature.

countercurrent heat exchange mechanism

If a tube carrying cool fluid runs adjacent to and in the same direction as one carrying warm fluid, heat will flow between them, and their temperatures will equalise. However, if the cool and warm fluids flow in opposite directions (countercurrent flow), and if the tubing is long enough, the cool fluid will warm to the temperature of the warm fluid and vice versa, a worthwhile gain over simple temperature equalisation (Fig. 7.12).

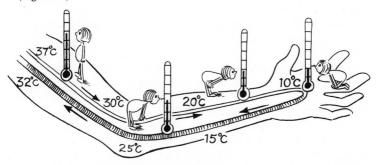

Fig. 7.12 *The countercurrent heat exchanger is a device which allows warm arterial blood entering a limb to progressively warm up the returning venous blood. Arterial blood reaching the hand may be 10°C, while the venous blood has been warmed to 32°C before entering the body.*

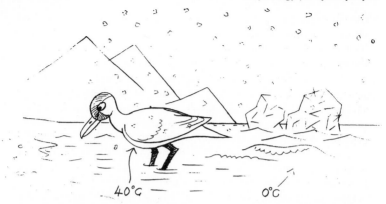

Fig. 7.13 Birds split their leg arteries and veins into many branches to give them an effective heat exchanger despite the shortness of their limbs.

The countercurrent heat exchanger is a cheap biological trick for reducing heat loss without reducing blood flow. In birds' legs, the artery and vein split into several small channels (called a *rete mirabile*, or marvellous net), making heat exchange very efficient despite their short leg length, and enabling them to wade cheerfully in near-freezing water with little heat loss.

In man, the major limb arteries and veins are adjacent to each other with flows in opposite directions and operate as countercurrent heat exchangers. Although not split as in birds, they are in close contact over a good length, making them a useful heat exchanger. In certain jobs, like that of commercial fishermen, bare hands are exposed to cold temperatures during winter. Thanks to the countercurrent heat exchange system, their hands and feet can be supplied with cooled arterial blood, which is warmed before returning to the body as venous blood at a temperature of around 35°C, having lost little heat. Many people, particularly women, complain of cold feet. This is actually a sign of the efficient operation of their heat exchanger. In cold weather, the veins on the surface of the forearm and on the back of the hand lie flat and almost disappear, another sign that the heat exchanger is operating, and that venous blood is returning to the body by deep veins running alongside arteries, and picking up heat from them on its way.

The countercurrent heat exchangers can be shut off to assist heat loss. In hot weather the venous blood from a limb returns to the body by a system of surface veins. On a hot day, these veins are full, standing out clearly visible on the inside surface of the forearms and the backs of the hands — evidence that the countercurrent heat exchanger has been turned off. Some seals and penguins cannot shut off -their countercurrent heat exchangers, and would suffer or even die in the relative warmth of a British winter.

sweat production

The signal to produce sweat comes from the hypothalamus, but depends on temperature information sent to it from the skin. As an example, assume that the temperature of the arterial blood has increased, and that the body needs to be cooled. If the skin temperature is low, the hypothalamus simply causes the skin blood flow to be increased, dissipating the excess heat passively.

However, if the blood flow to the skin rises, so will skin temperature, and may reach the point at which blood passing through the skin is inadequately cooled, and therefore cannot cool the body. The hypothalamus senses high skin temperature and initiates sweating, cooling the skin. Thus, sweat production is partly controlled by skin temperature, and partly by blood temperature. In exercise sweating diminishes if a fan is turned on to cool the skin, even if there is no change in the work rate, or in the temperature of arterial blood.

Although reduced, sweating does not stop in a cold climate. To some extent, sweating is initiated by the activity itself, regardless of any need for skin cooling. In very cold environments, sweating induced by activity can become a serious problem, wetting the clothing and impairing its insulating value. It is worth noting that Eskimos have fewer sweat glands on the trunk than do Caucasians, and perspire mainly on their faces. This is probably a hereditary adaptation, the result of thousands of years of arctic habitation.

Sweating is a powerful means of cooling. The evaporation of one litre of water takes up 550 kcal (2300 kJoules), or around 25% of a day's metabolic heat. So, in temperatures of over 32°C (90°F), where heat cannot be lost by convection, all of the metabolic heat must be lost by evaporation and over four litres would have to be evaporated daily simply to dissipate the heat produced by the normal metabolic rate. The maximum continuous rate of sweating is about one litre per hour, although sweating rates of two or three litres per hour have been recorded for short periods of time.

Sweating becomes less effective when the humidity is high and evaporation is hindered. Under such conditions sweat production is even more copious since the skin temperature fails to drop. Moreover, when sweat is produced at such high rates, it may drip uselessly off the body rather than evaporate, depleting body fluids without cooling properly (see Ch. 8).

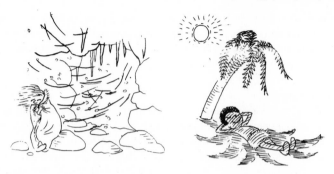

Fig. 7.14 We shelter from extremes of both heat and cold.

behavioural thermoregulation

Shelter is sought from extremes of both heat and cold. One may curl up to minimise surface area in the cold, or stretch out if heat loss is desired. Basking in the sun can be used to warm the skin and take up heat from a cool environment. Conversely, in countries such as Ghana or Sri Lanka, where temperatures are often very hot, basking or sunbathing is not popular.

Wind accelerates the rate of heat loss from the body in cold climates. In hot environments such as the Sahara, where air temperatures in excess of 50°C occur regularly, a great deal of heat can be gained by exposure to the wind. For this reason most animals, including man, shelter from the wind under both conditions of extreme heat and extreme cold.

Shelter for man includes clothing. Man has always worn protective clothing against both cold and hot environments. Thus, furs or thick woollens are worn by Eskimos and Laplanders. Desert dwellers such as the Bedouin of Arabia and the Tuareg of the Sahara, wear several layers of woollen garments to protect themselves against the extreme heat. They evaporate sweat into a "microclimate" beneath their robes, which is considerably cooler than the surrounding air.

Finally, if exercise is the cause of overheating, the behavioural instinct is to stop. Champions may exercise their will power to continue — occasionally causing themselves to suffer heat illness, or even death.

Summary

Man possesses a sophisticated thermoregulatory system which is capable of both warming and cooling the body to maintain a fairly constant "core" temperature (brain, abdomen and thorax) of 37°C. Core temperature normally falls during sleep and rises during exercise so that normal body temperature can range from a low of 36°C to a maximum of around 40°C. The limbs and skin generally remain cooler than the core, although the temperature of muscle in a working limb may be considerably warmer than 37°C.

Thermoregulation in exercise

In exercise, the amount of metabolic heat to be lost can increase by as much as sixteen times. Initially, the passive mechanisms for increasing heat dissipation are put into play. First, the flow of blood to the skin increases. With this influx of warm blood, the skin temperature rises. Indeed, although one may begin to exercise with cold hands, feet, ears and nose, within minutes the chill is usually gone.

Warming the skin has two effects. The warmer the skin, the more readily it can lose heat to the environment. However, as the skin temperature approaches blood temperature, the blood flowing through the skin is cooled less effectively. The rate of heat transfer depends upon both the temperature difference between the blood and the skin, and between the skin and the environment.

Since warming the skin makes it harder to cool the blood, the second stage of the thermoregulatory response is to cool the skin. Initially, this can be accomplished by removing clothing, or opening a window. On the sports field, after a warm-up, the sweatsuit is removed just before competition. As far as the athlete is concerned, warming up increases the temperature of the limb muscles. This allows them to develop a higher metabolic rate and increased power output, and by improving the speed of contraction, also helps co-ordination.*

The third stage occurs after the body has warmed up properly. The limbs are no longer cold, and body temperature has increased to its "working" value. This takes about five minutes, during which the body temperature will have risen to 38–40°C, depending on the work intensity and the environmental temperature.

capacity for heat dissipation

The maximum amount of sweat which can be produced by an unacclimatised person is about one litre per hour. The evaporation

---

* Warming up also reduces the chances of damage resulting from vigorous activity.

of one litre of water requires 550 kilocalories (kcal), so this rate of sweating can cope with a metabolic rate of approximately 9 kcal/min (550 kcal/60 min). This is the equivalent of using about two litres of oxygen per minute — hard but not maximum work, and the sort of work load which a young sedentary man might maintain over a thirty minute training session. This example assumes that 100% of the heat produced is dissipated by the evaporation of sweat. However, this would only be the case if the environmental temperature is so high (warmer than 32°C) that heat can only be lost by evaporation. Normally, some heat is lost to the environment by conduction and convection, economising on water. It is worth noting that sponsors and television interests often insist that sporting events be run in the afternoon, rather than in the cool of morning which would have been the athletes' or the physiologists' choice.

During hard work, skin blood flow can increase to around two litres per minute. With a temperature gradient of 6°C between the skin and arterial blood, $6 \times 2 = 12$ kcal/min can be transferred to the skin. This amount of heat is equivalent to an oxygen consumption of around 2.5 litres per minute, or greater than the continuous work rate of which an untrained man would be capable. Thus, the ability to produce sweat and the ability to deliver heat to the skin are usually adequate to cope with the demands of continuous hard work under realistic climatic conditions.* However, trained athletes are able to generate enough heat to tax their thermoregulation systems fully. In a marathon, they have the determination to run long enough, and in high enough temperatures, to ensure that dehydration can become a serious problem (see Ch. 8).

Heat acclimatisation or training to cope with heat

Heat acclimatisation is achieved by simply carrying out a normal endurance training programme under conditions of high environmental temperature. As with any physiological system, training depends upon repeated, high intensity use. Since the development of heat acclimatisation involves training in an activity, some of the

---

* Although the skin blood flow can be as high as 4 l/min, during hard work, demand for blood flow by other tissues limits it to about 2 l/min (Ch. 6, Fig. 7.26).

reported effects may be due to the inevitable improvement in physical fitness which must also occur.

Some heat acclimatisation does occur during training at moderate temperatures. This is because copious amounts of sweat are produced, and a high rate of blood flow to the skin is required, even at 20°C. In fact, if possible it is more sensible to train under conditions of moderate warmth initially. This is because an athlete from a cool climate will initially have a low tolerance for working in the heat, resulting in early fatigue or collapse. This lack of endurance may result in a "detraining" effect.

Heat acclimatisation has two basic effects. The first of these is improved cooling capacity. Thus the heat acclimatised individual can dissipate more metabolic heat, or tolerate work at a higher environmental temperature than an unacclimatised person. Secondly, endurance in the heat is improved so that after acclimatisation one can work longer in a hot environment before fatigue or collapse occurs. Some of these responses are related to changes in fluid balance and they will be mentioned briefly here and discussed later (Ch. 8).

skin blood flow
The volume of blood which can be sent to the skin increases so that more heat can be delivered to the surface of the body for dissipation. This allows the acclimatised individual to tolerate moderate work under conditions of extreme heat. Under sprint conditions, skin blood flow competes with the demand from working muscles, and it is unlikely that the maximum rate of skin blood flow is ever realised. In any case, during intense but brief duration work, the heat produced is simply stored in the body as a rise in temperature for dissipation later.

Note: By itself, an improved skin blood flow would be of limited use unless it is also accompanied by an increased rate of sweat production.

sweating rate
Sweat production begins more quickly after the start of exercise in the acclimatised individual. Acclimatisation makes the temperature control system more sensitive to rising temperature so that the sweat glands are stimulated earlier in exercise. This is not really advantageous since the rate at which the body temperature

rises is similar after acclimatisation, and a rapid rise to the working temperature is also desirable since this speeds up metabolism.

Following acclimatisation, the volume of sweat produced increases. More sweat glands appear to be active, these are more sensitive to instructions from the brain, and on stimulation they can produce twice as much sweat as before. This allows the skin to be maintained at a lower temperature. Since the rate at which heat is brought to the skin is determined by the temperature difference between skin and the arterial blood, any rate of heat dissipation can be maintained with a smaller blood flow. Where an unacclimatised individual might have to devote 2 l/min of blood flow to heat dissipation, an acclimatised person may cope with less than 1.5 l/min, diverting the difference (5–10% of maximum cardiac output) to their working muscles, and gaining an improvement in performance.

Acclimatisation reduces the sodium content of sweat. This makes the sweat slightly easier to evaporate. However, the main effect is that dilution of the sweat helps preserve the volume of the circulation helping the heart to maintain a high cardiac output during exercise (see Ch. 6 and 8 for details).

body temperature
Body temperature during exercise rises less after acclimatisation. A combination of the ability to produce more sweat, to circulate more blood through skin and increased sensitivity of the temperature regulating centre results in the ability to maintain a lower body temperature. This means that either a higher work load can be undertaken in the heat or that a particular work load can be carried out under hotter environmental conditions without danger of collapse.

Since very high blood temperatures can cause confusion, under competitive conditions the heat acclimatised athlete maintains a lower brain temperature, and better muscle co-ordination than an unacclimatised competitor.

blood volume
As sweat is produced and lost from the body, the blood volume becomes smaller and more concentrated. Together, these changes make it more difficult to pump blood around the body and the output of the heart is progressively reduced. During heat acclima-

tisation the blood volume increases, but the volume of plasma increases by more than does the volume of red cells, so the blood becomes slightly dilute. Starting with a slightly larger volume of more dilute blood simply increases the amount of sweat which can be produced before the cardiac output drops to the point of interfering with performance. In short, endurance is improved (see p. 181).

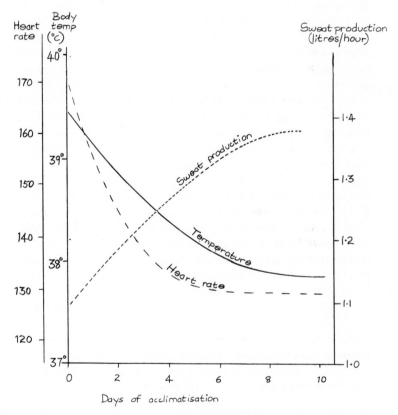

Fig. 7.16 In an experiment on heat acclimatisation, heart rates, body temperatures and the rate of sweat production were all measured after 100 minutes of walking at 49°C. The experiment itself was the subjects' only exposure to heat. A substantial improvement is seen within one week.

an example of heat acclimatisation

A group of untrained, but reasonably fit men were made to walk on a treadmill in a climatic chamber maintained at 49°C (very hot indeed) for periods of 100 minutes each day, for ten days. Their work load was moderate and set to require about one litre of oxygen per minute. This produced heat at the rate of 350 Watts, or four times the resting value.

On the first few days many of the men were unable to complete 100 minutes of work at this very high temperature. Figure 7.16 shows that their heart rates and rectal temperatures were very high. Within two days there was a marked improvement in their performance, and all the men were able to complete the task. After one week their sweat production had increased by 30% and their rectal temperature had dropped by 1.5°C. Most dramatic was the improvement in their heart rate. One week of acclimatisation to heat had reduced the heart rate at the end of 100 minutes of walking at 49°C to just 10% higher than it had been before training, when walking in a cool environment!

At the start of the experiment, sweat production was low, implying that skin temperature was high and that a large skin blood flow was required to dissipate heat. Even so, the body temperature at the end of exercise was high. After nine days of acclimatisation, sweating had increased, cooling the skin more effectively and reducing the volume of blood required for cooling. The reduction in heart rate shows how much less work was required of the heart, while the drop in body temperature shows that cooling was even more effective.

Summary

Heat acclimatisation is not just a problem for the athlete. In temperate countries with cool winters and hot summers, "heat waves" are associated with increases in mortality of over 30%. For the most part, it is the elderly who die, and circulatory failure is the cause of death. For these people, the effort of cooling clearly exceeds the capacity of their cardiovascular system. Interestingly, the first "heat wave" of the summer is responsible for most of these "excess" deaths. The development of heat acclimatisation presumably protects people from the effects of later spells of hot weather.

Only endurance athletes really need worry about heat acclimatisation. During the first ten minutes of exercise the body temperature is rising to its "working" value. For this reason, the ability to cool the body has little or no effect on sprint or middle distance performance. It is only after 15–20 minutes of work under hot climatic conditions that cooling becomes important because of increasing quantities of blood diverted to the skin. Any blood flow sent to the skin is not available to the working muscles and must diminish performance.

For the most part, the decrease in performance due to the need for cooling is slight, although probably important in the split-second world of athletics. However, the effect on endurance is of far greater practical importance. Acclimatisation to work under hot climatic conditions can achieve substantial gains in endurance. In properly acclimatised individuals, endurance in the heat is only slightly poorer than it would be under cool conditions.

The question of heat acclimatisation is intimately linked to the volume of fluid lost in sweat and to the body's ability to cope with the decrease in cardiovascular performance which this causes (Ch. 8).

CHAPTER EIGHT

Fluid balance in exercise

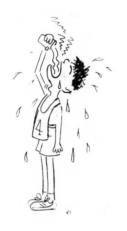

The body can sweat several litres of water in a few hours. Yet the loss of just one litre of water from the circulating blood volume can partially disable the cardiovascular system and considerably reduce its performance. A greater loss can cause collapse and hyperthermia (a dangerously high body temperature).

When working in a hot environment, a person's work output is unimpaired at first and similar to what can be achieved at lower temperatures. With time, performance drops off more rapidly under hot conditions than in a cool environment. Under hot climatic conditions, endurance is closely linked to fluid balance. In simple terms, on a hot day many marathon runners are stopped by their water loss, and by the overheating which accompanies it.

Work in the heat — time to exhaustion

An experiment was carried out in which a group of sedentary volunteers were made to work to exhaustion on exercise bicycles. They pedalled at a load equivalent to 70% of their maximum work capacity. This experiment was repeated under both hot and cold environmental conditions, and the time to exhaustion (taken when the set work load could no longer be sustained) was noted. At an environmental temperature of 20°C, their endurance was 72 minutes. At 33°C, this was halved to 33 minutes.

Clearly, endurance is markedly reduced at high temperatures.

When the same subjects were given water to drink during the experiment, their time to exhaustion in the heat was increased by over 20%. In the low temperature trial, less sweat was formed and fluid loss played a relatively small role in exhaustion. Here, drinking water increased the subjects' endurance by only 6%.

Some questions

Why is endurance reduced in a hot environment, and why does water replacement improve it?

Where does the water to form sweat come from, and what effect does water loss have on the cardiovascular system?

How large are the body's water resources, and how long can they cool properly?

How easy is it to replace lost fluid, and how quickly can this be done? Can this be improved by training?

Can the body store water in anticipation of sweating?

Can an athlete rehydrate effectively during exercise?

The answers to these questions emerge from an understanding of the body's fluid compartments and the way these are regulated.

The body's fluids form separate compartments

Approximately 60% of the weight of a man and 50% of the weight of a woman is water (Fig. 8.2). Fat tissue excludes water and very lean people may be as much as 80% water, while the obese may have less than 40%. The internal fat deposits (around the heart, kidneys, etc.) increase with age. For this reason, the elderly tend to have more fat and less water than the young. Despite the increase in total fat, the amount of subcutaneous fat (fat just under the skin) declines with age, giving rise to the skin wrinkling which is characteristic of the elderly. Subcutaneous fat deposits make a woman's skin feel softer than a man's, while specific regions with sexually determined fat deposits give women their distinctive shape. These deposits make women fatter and less "watery" on average than men (see also Ch. 10).

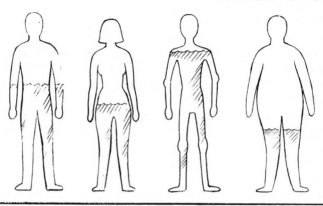

Fig. 8.2 The body's water content depends on fatness.

There are 45 litres (79 pints or 10 imperial gallons) of water in a 70 kg male and 30 litres (53 pints or 6.6 gallons) in a 60 kg female (Fig. 8.3). Two thirds of this water is inside the body's cells, and is called "intracellular". The remainder is located outside the cells, and is thus termed "extracellular". The extracellular and intracellular fluid compartments are separated from one another by the cell membranes. These are "semi-permeable" and prevent the passage of certain dissolved substances while allowing others to cross freely. Cell membranes do not normally allow

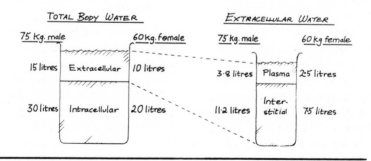

Fig. 8.3 Part of the body's water is inside (intracellular) cells and part is outside (extracellular). The extracellular water can be subdivided into the portion which is in the circulation (plasma) and that which is outside the blood vessels and heart (interstitial fluid).

sodium or protein to pass, while water and potassium can move across readily (see p. 8). For this reason, the composition of the intracellular and the extracellular fluids differ markedly.

Intracellular fluid is a solution of salts containing potassium as its major positive ion (when salts dissolve in water they split up into positively and negatively charged particles called ions) while the negative charges are carried by the cell proteins. The extracellular fluid has sodium as its major positive ion while negative charges are carried by the chloride and the bicarbonate ions. The difference in composition between the two compartments is created by membrane pumping systems which transport certain ions into and out of the cells, and is maintained by the cell membranes.

Osmotic pressure and the blood flow

The extracellular compartment consists of the blood plasma (three litres) and the interstitial fluid or the solution bathing cells, which is about four times larger. The compositions of these subcompartments are very similar, except that there is protein dissolved in plasma, while the interstitial fluid has little.

The plasma and interstitial fluid are separated by the porous, leaky wall of the capillary vessels. This allows most materials in the extracellular fluid to pass freely, barring only protein, the red blood cells, and platelets (which promote blood clotting). The circulatory system is pressurised by the work of the heart, while the interstitial fluid is near zero pressure. The pressure within the circulation causes fluid to ooze out of the capillaries near their arterial end (Fig. 8.4). Since the capillary wall is not permeable to protein, this is left behind in the capillary, and protein concentration increases as fluid is lost. Meanwhile, the hydrostatic pressure the heart has given to the blood drops along the length of the capillary. Eventually, osmotic pressure overcomes decreasing hydrostatic pressure and returns most of the lost fluid to the circulation at the venous end.

Osmotic pressure develops across a semi-permeable membrane whenever the solutions on either side have different strengths or concentrations (Fig. 8.5). Osmotic pressure causes the solvent to flow (by osmosis) through the membrane, from the dilute (weaker) solution to the more concentrated (stronger) solution. Osmotic

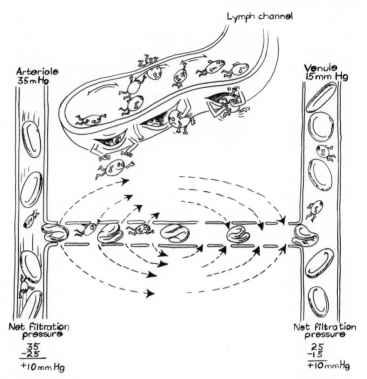

Arteriole
35 m Hg

Lymph channel

Venule
15 mm Hg

Net filtration
pressure

35
-25
+10 mm Hg

Net filtration
pressure

25
-15
+10 mm Hg

Fig. 8.4 Capillaries are porous so that plasma oozes out into the inter-stitial fluid (Fig. 8.3) at their arterial end. However, the capillaries do not permit the plasma proteins to leak out and they exert an osmotic pressure which brings back the leaked fluid at the venous end of the capillary. Any protein which managed to escape is scavenged by the lymphatic vessels.

movement is always in the direction which tends to equalise the concentrations across the membrane. The amount of osmotic pressure developed depends on the difference in concentration of the solutions on either side of the membrane.

Plasma contains dissolved protein, which cannot cross the capillary wall, while the interstitial fluid has little. This protein exerts an osmotic pressure which encourages any water which has escaped from the circulation to return to the plasma (Fig. 8.4). The correct concentration of protein in plasma is partly responsible for maintaining the normal volume of blood.

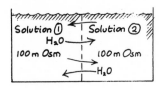

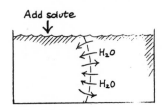

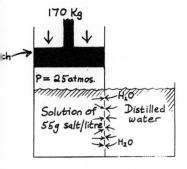

Fig. 8.5 *Water moves freely across the membrane, but the volume of flow in both directions is the same. If a solute which cannot cross the membrane is added to one compartment, the volume of water moving into that compartment becomes greater than the volume going the other way, creating an osmotic pressure. In theory this can be measured by applying enough pressure to one side of the apparatus to prevent osmotic movement. Such an apparatus can be used to desalinate sea water.*

In starvation and in pregnancy the concentration of plasma protein drops, and oedema results (swelling caused by the accumulation of interstitial fluid as water leaks out of the plasma). If the capillaries are physically damaged (by a high speed cricket ball or ice hockey puck), plasma proteins leak out into the interstitial space decreasing the concentration gradient across the capillary and the osmotic pressure. This causes local oedema. If the damage is severe enough to allow red blood cells to leak out as well, a colourful bruise will form. When this happens, the lymphatic system gradually picks up the leaked protein and fluid, returning it to the circulation.

some examples of osmosis at work in the body
1. Effects of drinking water:
   Water is absorbed from the gut into the blood and the extracellular fluid, whose concentrations are thus reduced. Water flows down its osmotic gradient into the cells until their concentration is the same as that of the surrounding fluid.
   Potassium cannot easily leave the cells because it cannot take its negatively charged companion, the

protein, along. Nor can it trade places with sodium, which is unable to cross cell membranes.

1. Add water

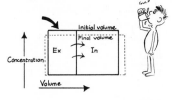

The net effect is that both compartments become larger and are diluted.

2. Effects of eating salt:

Salt, or sodium chloride, is absorbed into the blood and the extracellular fluid, concentrating both compartments. Since sodium cannot enter cells (and is actively pumped out of them), water flows from the cells.

2. Add NaCl

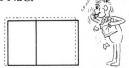

The net effect is that both compartments become more concentrated, and the extracellular compartment increases in volume at the expense of intracellular water. This cell shrinkage also stimulates thirst.

3. Drinking water following (2):

Consumption of salty food causes thirst. The amount of water consumed afterwards tends to be just enough to bring body fluids back to their normal concentration.

3. Add isotonic NaCl solution

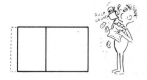

The net effect is therefore that of having drunk a volume of isosmotic (normal body concentration) fluid. There is no change in the concentration of the body fluids, but the extracellular volume increases, while cell volume remains unchanged.

4. Effect of losing salt:

The sweat of most people on a normal diet and not acclimatised to hot environments has the same concentration as the extracellular fluid. Sweating therefore simply reduces extracellular volume.

4. Lose NaCl

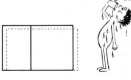

Fig. 8.6

176

Drinking water alone cannot replace the lost sweat because this dilutes the extracellular fluid, and much of the added water is transferred osmotically into cells.

Drinking water after sweating simply has the net effect of losing salt, shrinking the extracellular fluid, expanding the intracellular fluid, and diluting both.

In exercise, both water and salt are lost

The above examples show most of the changes in body fluids which can be experienced by people in the course of their normal daily activities. In exercise, sweat is produced for cooling. For short periods of time, sweat can be produced at the rate of four litres per hour, although one litre per hour is more usual in long term activity. The loss of this sweat means that the body is depleted of water and salt (sodium chloride), shrinking the extracellular fluid compartment (case 4. above).

Usually, the food intake, the kidney, and the thirst mechanism work together to maintain the size and composition of the body's fluid compartments. However, in competitive exercise the kidney barely functions or may even be shut down. (Its blood supply is temporarily diverted to the working muscles.) Although the kidney's regulatory function may be lost for a time, this at least prevents either water or solutes from leaving the body in the urine.

In track and field meets there are opportunities to consume water or food between events. Although athletes may drink at this time, few consume the one or two litres of fluid each hour which might be necessary for complete fluid replacement. Likewise, not many active participants consume anything other than sweets or chocolate at athletic meetings. More substantial food would make them feel full and less like performing. The salt content of such confections is low and does not begin to replace what has been lost.

The extracellular volume cannot usually be maintained during an athletic meet or a game such as tennis or football. Often this does not matter because fluid depletion probably has little effect on performance if activity is limited to one or two hours and some fluid replacement is possible in breaks. In any case, moderate dehydration has less effect than would a litre of sports drink sloshing around in the stomach. Depending on the intensity of exercise, the rate of blood flow through the digestive tract may be so reduced that if food or water is consumed, little may be absorbed.

Control of osmotic pressure

The concentration of the blood is monitored by an organ in the brain called the "osmoreceptor" which can detect changes of less than one per cent in the osmotic pressure. Drinking dilutes the body fluids. The osmoreceptors sense this, suppressing thirst and discouraging the drinking of more water.

The osmoreceptor also produces antidiuretic hormone (ADH), which causes the kidney to conserve water by producing a small volume of concentrated urine — as little as half a litre per day. After drinking water, the ADH production stops and its concentration in the blood declines. Within twenty minutes the kidney is able to increase the urine volume. If enough water has been drunk, there may be no ADH in the blood, and urine formation can be as high as one litre per hour, rapidly clearing the ingested water from the body and restoring normal osmotic pressure.

Normally, the operation of the system is precise, and the consumption of water is rapidly followed by the excretion of a similar volume of water. Interestingly, alcohol specifically inhibits the osmoreceptor's production of ADH, causing the kidney to produce large volumes of dilute urine. In effect, if beer is consumed, a larger volume of water will be excreted in the urine. This, in turn, leads to the dehydration and thirst which is characteristic of (and may be the cause of) a hangover.

If the body is progressively dehydrated, the osmoreceptor produces increasing quantities of ADH, reducing urine volume and increasing its concentration to a maximum of about four times that of plasma. Simultaneously, another mechanism activated by the osmoreceptor gives rise to the sensation of thirst. Depending on other claims for our attention at the time, we will eventually be forced to drink.

Control of volume

The mechanisms which control the extracellular fluid volume, and blood volume in particular, are more complex than those in charge of the osmotic pressure. Volume is not easy for the body to measure. Instead, various pressure measurements are used to indicate volume. These are made principally in the large veins near the heart and in the heart itself. The degree of stretch to which these organs are subject is a good index of the venous pressure, and hence volume. The kidney appears to use the difference between systolic and diastolic arterial pressure (see Ch. 6) as an independent index of blood volume, and to regulate the hormone aldosterone, which controls sodium excretion.

If blood volume is reduced, even in the absence of any change in concentration which might be detected by the osmoreceptor (for example, by haemorrhage), ADH production will be stimulated, reducing the kidney's loss of water. This response is initiated by volume sensing devices. The volume sensors also stimulate aldosterone production reducing the rate at which the body loses salt (sodium chloride) by the kidney, sweat glands (see p. 186), intestine, and saliva.

However, the kidney cannot create water and salt. Following a volume loss, the drinking of water and food consumption (containing salt) are the only way to rectify the deficit. The aldosterone controlled retention of sodium and chloride within the extracellular fluid is the necessary accompaniment to the water retention encouraged by ADH. Together, the two hormones collaborate to increase the volume of the extracellular fluid.

Sweat production and fluid balance

The water for sweat production is extracted from the blood supply by the sweat glands, and depends on an adequate flow of blood to the skin. This water is removed from the plasma, affecting the ability of the cardiovascular system to pump blood (below). Since plasma volume is three to four litres, only a limited amount of sweat may be formed without seriously depleting blood volume, unless the water loss can be shared with other body fluid compartments.

Human sweat contains no protein (horses' sweat does, causing

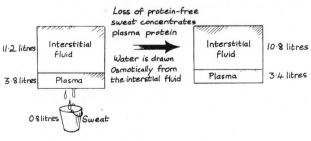

Fig. 8.7

179

it to foam). Removal of plasma water to form sweat raises the concentration of protein in the plasma, and the plasma osmotic pressure. This brings water in from the interstitial fluid (Fig. 8.7). Thus, if one litre of sweat is produced, approximately half of this comes from the plasma volume and half from the interstitial fluid. (If not for this mechanism, a larger proportion of the sweat volume would have to come from the plasma.)

Other factors also play a role in determining what proportion of the volume of sweat produced is drawn from the plasma. Heat acclimatisation and diet have important effects on this, and hence on endurance in hot climates. This will be discussed in more detail below (pp. 184, 186).

Heat dissipation and fluid balance in exercise

can water be stored?
True water storage is not possible since any extra water taken in is rapidly lost in the urine. However, physical activity directly stimulates the production of ADH. So if water is taken just prior to exercise, the expected increase in urine volume will not occur, and this water will have been "stored" for use in thermoregulation. It is probably not possible to store more than one litre in this way, and even that might make an athlete feel uncomfortable.

sweat production, fluid balance and cardiovascular performance
The blood volume is a key factor governing cardiovascular performance. However, the cardiovascular system's capacity is elastic, and the system is quite tolerant of volume changes. It will accept additional volume (for example: drinking a quantity of beer) by relaxing the veins so that the venous pressure barely changes. Fortunately, the kidney's ability to excrete water (it can produce well over one litre per hour — continuously!) comfortably exceeds man's ability to drink. Disease apart (heart or renal disease) an overfilled cardiovascular system is seldom a problem for very long.

The cardiovascular system can still function when underfilled (Fig. 8.8). A low blood volume drops venous pressure, reducing the ability of the heart to fill (p. 125). The smooth muscle in the walls of the veins then constricts them to maintain venous pressure so that blood can continue to return to the heart. However, venous constriction also increases the resistance to blood flow in the veins. At first venous constriction improves the rate at which

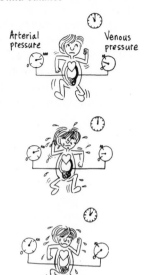

Fig. 8.8 During prolonged exercise, a large volume of sweat may be lost. As fluid is lost blood volume is reduced, and venous pressure tends to fall. Initially, constriction of the veins maintains venous pressure, and arterial pressure does not fall (see Ch. 6, p. 125). If enought fluid is lost, the heart cannot fill properly and arterial pressure drops, terminating activity abruptly.

the blood returns to the heart. A limit is reached when the beneficial effects of boosting venous pressure are cancelled by increasing resistance to flow. At rest this starts to happen after more than one litre of blood volume has been lost; in exercise, half a litre is a more likely limit since the demands on the heart are that much greater.

The removal of fluid to produce sweat increases the concentration of both protein and cells in the plasma, increasing the blood viscosity. Together, venous constriction and rising viscosity combine to increase the resistance to blood flow in the veins, making it even more difficult for the heart to fill. In an attempt to maintain cardiac output, the pulse rate increases as stroke volume goes down and a rapid pulse is a typical symptom of both haemorrhage and dehydration. In fact, the loss of water by sweating hampers cardiac output far more than would the loss of a similar volume through haemorrhage.

At rest, the loss of over 1.5 litres of blood volume results in collapse (called shock — see p. 124) and threatens survival. Collapse from shock does not occur during exercise. Instead, when fluid volume drops enough to affect cardiac output, athletic performance must fall as well. If motivation is very high the athlete may maintain speed for a time while the body "economises" on blood flow to the skin and on sweat production. This soon results in severe overheating called "explosive heat rise" (below).

Even a modest degree of dehydration will have a clear effect on physical performance. Although its effect varies between individuals and also depends on the circumstances, a total water loss equivalent to 2% of the body weight (about 1.5 litres) may reduce endurance by 20% and maximum oxygen consumption (which depends on the output of the heart) by 10%.

deliberate water loss
Athletes may deliberately dehydrate themselves to meet target weights. This is particularly common among boxers and wrestlers who fight in specific weight categories. Although several hours might elapse between the weigh-in and the actual competition, these athletes often fight in a dehydrated state, with the expected consequences for performance (see p. 204).

A variety of methods is used by athletes to lose weight just before the weigh-in. These include sweating without drinking, the use of diuretic agents which greatly increase the urine volume, induction of vomiting, and the use of laxatives. All of these can seriously disturb the acid-alkaline balance of the body, and should not be encouraged. If a boxer or wrestler consistently has trouble meeting his target weight, it is likely that he really ought to be fighting at a higher weight.

Another group of sportsmen who need to meet target weights, and who may dehydrate themselves for this purpose are racing jockeys. In this case, their performance is unlikely to be affected by the procedure!

Cardiovascular performance, thermoregulation and explosive heat rise

In a hot environment, rectal temperature increases steadily as dehydration proceeds because the sweat production drops. Rectal temperature rises to 39°C when the water deficit reaches 10% of body weight, even in a person at rest. If moderate work is performed, the same body temperature is achieved at only 6% dehydration. Water loss clearly limits the amount of work which can be carried out in a hot climate.

If the environmental temperature is high enough, progressive dehydration during exercise eventually causes "explosive heat rise".

This is a failure of regulation in which the body temperature rises rapidly, and to a high value. Its immediate cause is a decrease in cardiovascular performance due to the reduction in blood volume and a drop in the cardiac output. This eventually makes it impossible to send an adequate flow of blood to the skin, either for cooling or for sweat production. The higher the work rate, the sooner explosive heat rise will occur.

On the other hand, overheating, distress and collapse can be delayed or even prevented by drinking. Experiments have shown that during treadmill walking at high temperature, drinking water at half-hour intervals increased endurance by 25% (Fig. 8.9). Guided by their thirst, the subjects drank less than half the volume of water they were losing as sweat, and eventually succumbed to overheating. However, when they were forced to drink the same volume of water that they had lost as sweat during the previous half-hour, there was no overheating at all. Their endurance was now determined by fatigue, and not by the distress and collapse of explosive heat rise.

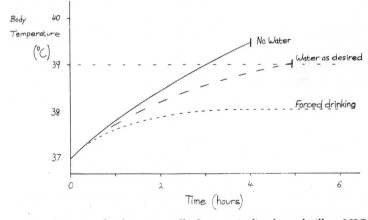

Fig. 8.9 *A group of volunteers walked on an inclined treadmill at 38°C. Without drinking, temperature rose steadily and endurance was limited to four hours. Drinking every half-hour, temperature still rose but endurance was increased. When the volunteers were forced to drink a volume equal to the sweat they had produced during the previous half-hour, body temperature remained low and the experiment was stopped with no sign of heat exhaustion.*

Importance of salt in the sweat

sweating in the unacclimatised individual — salty sweat
The salt concentration in sweat ranges from a high value similar
to that in plasma down to nearly zero. An unacclimatised person
with a normal "western" diet containing 10 to 15 grams of salt
daily, produces sweat with a great deal of salt. Most people, after
half an hour of sweating, have experienced stinging as sweat runs
into their eyes (and wear sweat bands to prevent this). The irritation is caused by the highly concentrated salt solution left behind
when sweat evaporates. On occasion, the skin may even become
gritty with the crystallised salt.

In an unacclimatised person, the fluid leaving the sweat glands
initially has the same salt concentration as blood, but contains no

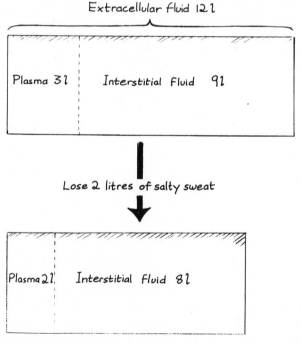

Extracellular fluid 12 l

Plasma 3 l | Interstitial Fluid 9 l

Lose 2 litres of salty sweat

Plasma 2 l | Interstitial Fluid 8 l

*Fig. 8.10 The loss of two litres of salty (the same concentration as
plasma) sweat is shared equally between the plasma volume and the much
larger interstitial fluid (see also Fig. 8.7).*

protein. The loss of this protein-free fluid increases the plasma
protein concentration, drawing water into the plasma by osmosis
protein concentration, drawing water into the plasma by osmosis
from the interstitial fluid. This means that the water loss is not
borne entirely by the plasma volume, but is shared with the much
larger interstitial fluid volume. Typically, half of the volume of
sweat produced comes from the plasma, and the rest is from the
interstitial fluid (Figs. 8.7 & 8.10).

limits of sweating
Thus, the loss of one litre of sweat reduces blood volume by 0.5
litre, the practical maximum which still permits a reasonably high
cardiac output to be pumped. This is equivalent to dissipating by
evaporation all of the heat that a "three-hour" marathon runner
might produce in thirty minutes*, a rate of 1.5 litres of sweat each
hour. Fortunately runners can usually lose heat by other means as
well, because 1.5 litres per hour represents a high rate of sweat
production which cannot be long sustained. In any case, drinking
is allowed and even encouraged during a marathon.

Continued formation of sweat without fluid replacement so
reduces cardiac output that high levels of physical activity would
be rapidly curtailed (Fig. 8.8). The survival limit is reached when
the plasma volume is reduced by less than two litres, implying that
less than four litres of sweat may be produced before replacement

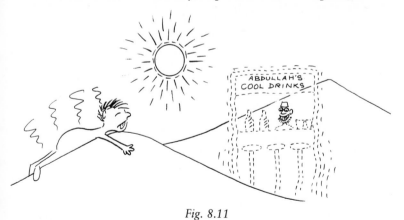

Fig. 8.11

* 1 hour of running costs 1100 kcal (p. 37) and evaporation of 1 l water dissipates
550 kcal (p. 152).

is required. In fact more sweat can be produced, and losses of just over five litres (7% of the body weight) have been recorded after eight hours of walking in desert conditions at 35°C. The maximum tolerable dehydration is 10% of the body weight, but then the very reduced cardiac output is able to support no activity, not even walking. Since marathons are run at speed, often at high temperatures, and last two to four hours, the body clearly has resources over and above the extracellular fluid. What are these?

where does sweat come from?
About one litre of salty sweat must be produced before the volume loss can be detected (the volume sensing system is quite slow). The plasma concentration of aldosterone (the hormone responsible for sodium or salt conservation) increases. Under the influence of aldosterone, the sodium content of sweat (and urine, saliva, and faeces) is substantially reduced. As dilute sweat is produced, the extracellular fluid from which it has been extracted becomes more concentrated (Fig. 8.12). This increase in concentration draws water, by osmosis, out of the cells and into the extracellular fluid.

Thus, although most of the initial litre of sweat produced comes from the extracellular fluid (interstitial fluid plus plasma) part of the later, dilute sweat production is drawn from the very large intracellular reservoir (below). From the viewpoint of endurance, it is a pity that so much of the early sweat must be taken from the plasma where it has such a negative effect on performance. It is, however, possible to improve on this.

sweating in the heat acclimatised individual — salt is precious
A respectable degree of heat acclimatisation can be achieved by living and working in a hot climate for about one week. During the first few days, salty sweat (concentration similar to plasma) is produced. After an initial salt loss (provided that this loss is only partly replaced), the adrenal glands increase their secretion of aldosterone. As long as more salt is lost in the sweat than is taken in the diet, the secretion of aldosterone steadily rises. If enough of this hormone is produced, sodium can virtually vanish from the sweat and urine. However, this is unlikely to occur in people taking a liberally salted "Western" diet.

As explained previously, producing a dilute sweat allows some of the water for further sweat production to be drawn from the

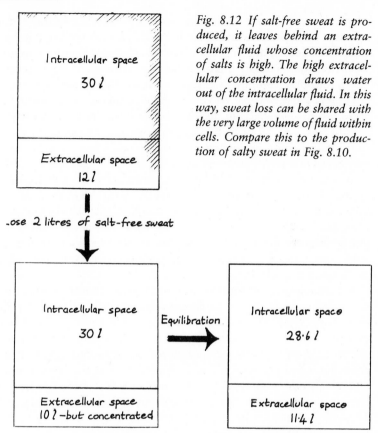

Fig. 8.12 *If salt-free sweat is produced, it leaves behind an extracellular fluid whose concentration of salts is high. The high extracellular concentration draws water out of the intracellular fluid. In this way, sweat loss can be shared with the very large volume of fluid within cells. Compare this to the production of salty sweat in Fig. 8.10.*

body's cells, improving endurance. Groups of people living far from the sea in equatorial Brazil, Papua New Guinea, and Botswana who have no access to salt, are able to produce nearly salt-free sweat. There are anecdotal reports of !Kung San ("Kalahari Bushmen" — the "!" denotes a click in their language) hunters jogging after wounded game animals for 8-9 hours without water at temperatures of over 30°C. If true, this represents a prodigious feat of endurance. These hunters also seem to have a remarkable ability to rapidly rehydrate themselves (see p. 189).

salt may be precious, but it's also cheap — to salt or not to salt?
Acute salt loss may cause muscle cramps, dizziness, or fainting.

This commonly occurs in unacclimatised individuals during their first two days of working in the heat. Taking salt tablets rapidly replenishes losses, and relieves the symptoms. On the other hand, well trained athletes are often partly heat acclimatised. This comes about through copious sweating, whether they train in a hot environment or not. Moreover, in athletes the administration of extra salt has no effect on their performance in hot environments.

However, salt supplementation prevents the development of a salt deficit. Issuing salt tablets used to be common practice during military manoeuvres in tropical climates. Although salt supplements may alleviate the immediate symptoms of deficit, they delay acclimatisation and prevent its full development. The practice has now been largely abandoned, partly because salt tablets tend to cause nausea and may irritate the stomach and intestine. Although salt tablets are out of fashion today, beverages containing "electrolytes" (table salt mainly), often labelled sports drinks, are actively promoted (see p. 190).

An acclimatised person taking no salt supplements produces a dilute sweat which leaves the blood relatively concentrated. Fluid then moves readily from the intracellular space into the plasma by osmosis. Since the intracellular space is large, the ability to obtain water from the cells to produce sweat can make an appreciable contribution to endurance, and performance. On the other hand, individuals with a salty diet lose appreciable quantities of salt in their sweat leaving the blood concentration relatively unchanged. The amount of plasma replenishment from cell water in such people is small, reducing their endurance.

Rehydration — thirst and drinking after dehydration

Thirst is induced in two ways. Decreasing the body's extracellular fluid volume initially has little effect, but thirst is powerfully stimulated once the deficit exceeds 5%. More commonly, thirst is controlled by changes in the concentration of the body fluids. If their concentration increases, thirst is stimulated. If they are diluted, thirst is suppressed.

After producing salty sweat (but never more concentrated than plasma), the plasma volume is reduced but its concentration is largely unchanged. If the volume decrease is small, then thirst is only weakly stimulated. Drinking water then dilutes the plasma, suppresses thirst, and limits the rate at which rehydration can proceed. In practice, even a very thirsty individual will find it hard to consume more than one litre of water at a time (try it!). More water can be taken after eating, when salt has been taken in with the food. Some people claim that, after sweating, they crave salty foods or salt and put more of it on their food. (Herbivorous animals are known to have a specific salt appetite, but its existence in man is still controversial.)

In subjects who are exercising steadily, even if water or other beverages are provided, it is almost impossible for them to drink enough to prevent some degree of dehydration. The dilution of body fluids caused by water intake ensures that the sensation of thirst always lags behind their water deficit. Attempts to increase water ingestion during exercise by providing beverages with added salt have not been particularly successful (see below).

However, if a dilute sweat is produced, the plasma becomes concentrated. In this situation a larger volume of water can be consumed before the dilution of plasma suppresses thirst and drinking, and rehydration can proceed more rapidly. This is seen clearly in animals that pant. Very little salt is lost in panting because evaporation occurs internally in the mouth and respiratory passages, leaving the body fluids concentrated and increasing the thirst sensation. Most panting animals such as dogs, donkeys or goats are capable of drinking most of the volume lost during thermoregulation at a single sitting — and with astonishing precision. Donkeys weighing just 25% more than a man, experimentally dehydrated by desert walks, have been observed drinking over twenty litres in under three minutes! This huge intake simply dilutes their body fluids back to their normal concentration.

The !Kung San or "Kalahari Bushmen" have long been known for their ability to rehydrate very rapidly. These hunter-gatherers live in a hot desert environment where surface water is scarce. They rely on underground caches stored in ostrich egg shells, and on watery roots for emergency supplies of drinking water. Their traditional diet is composed of nearly salt-free nuts and roots. The small amount of salt they consume is obtained from the meat in their diet, and they produce an almost salt-free sweat. Their body fluids become concentrated as they sweat, and drinking simply dilutes them back to a normal concentration. Individual San weighing 55 kg have been observed consuming five litres of water at one sitting, achieving nearly complete and very rapid rehydration.

Commercial sports drinks — rehydration v. energy supplement

Additional fluid intake is absorbed best when dilute, and NOT as a heavily sweetened beverage. Even fluids with the same concentration as blood are not absorbed as well as plain water. In any case, the maximum rate of fluid absorption in a working endurance athlete is less than 800 ml/hr. (Absorption is limited by the great reduction in blood supply to the digestive tract during exercise — Ch. 6.) This is slower than their maximum rate of sweat production! So complete replacement is generally not possible. Athletes are also very likely to complain that their performance is hampered by large quantities of liquid in their stomach!

Manufacturers have not been slow to spot a market for rehydration beverages and to capitalise on it. Accordingly, some of the research in this area has been commercially sponsored, and may be biased or even unreliable. The stated aim is to provide a drink which is: (a) rapidly absorbed, (b) provides some of the lost salt, and (c) replaces some of the carbohydrate consumed during activity. However, absorption is fastest when the beverage is considerably less concentrated than the body fluids. Clearly, this limitation means that it is only realistic to replace a small part of the lost salt. This is particularly true when recalling that, in endurance exercise at high temperatures, voluntary drinking does not replace the fluid lost (see above p. 189).

Attempts to replace some of the carbohydrate used during exercise have also come up against problems. The presence of sugar in the stomach retards emptying, and this greatly slows intestinal fluid absorption. A 10% sugar solution is absorbed at half the speed of plain water. Traditional carbonated soft drinks (non-diet) vary between 8% and 13% sugar. Certain American beverages marketed as sports drinks contain only 5% sugar (eg: "Gatorade", "Instant Replay"), but even these markedly retard fluid absorption. Moreover, an athlete drinking one 300 ml can of such a beverage receives just 60 kcal — enough to sustain five minutes of cross-country running, or three minutes of competitive running. Thus, these beverages only supply a very small amount of energy, but this does not stop them from selling well.

The desire to replace fluid must be traded off against the replacement of energy. However, with respect to the needs of the athlete, neither can be replaced completely.

Another recent approach has been to supply the energy as large polymer molecules which are chains of sugar molecules. Because these large molecules exert far less osmotic pressure than would a similar weight of simple sugar, they can be administered in larger quantities and still allow reasonably fast absorption of both nutrients and water. The effects of three test beverages: 750 ml of water, a 4% glucose solution, and a 20% solution of glucose polymer, have been tested on the exercise performance of volunteers. All of these were made up as beverages with similar taste and appearance. Exhaustion occurred at 140 minutes drinking water, at 160 minutes drinking 4% glucose, and at 180 minutes drinking the 20% glucose polymer preparation, suggesting that the polymer had been beneficial.

It is however worth keeping in mind that few athletes will wish to compete with almost one litre of fluid in their stomachs before the event. It may be that, particularly in the case of a runner, the extra weight of fluid may slow them down even as endurance is improved, yielding little real advantage. If instead the fluid was taken as several small drinks, slowing down to drink would probably slow the runner even more.

Of potentially greater interest is the effect of sugary beverages or carbohydrate foods taken immediately before an event on the metabolism of the athlete. To the casual observer, this should boost blood glucose and increase the available supply of energy for exercise. However, taking sugar or starch in any form promotes insulin secretion. (This hormone lowers the blood glucose concentration by promoting its metabolism and storage as glycogen.) However, it also slows the mobilisation of fats, forcing the body to use carbohydrate instead. Anything which causes insulin to be secreted just before endurance competition actually decreases endurance. If you must consume something, make sure you leave at least thirty minutes before competition begins, allowing insulin to return to normal by start time.

Dressing the part

Today, wearing a full Victorian costume in the tropics would be considered insane, particularly if the wearer also engaged in energetic activity. Yet the Victorians walked the length and breadth of Africa elegantly dressed in woollen coats, high collars, and even multiple petticoats. Although their attire looks quite unsuitable to us, it evidently had little effect on their performance — of course, they were not competing.

It is interesting to note what well-dressed Tuareg and Bedouin wear in their Saharan and Arabian desert homes. Their customary dress consists of multiple layers of long woollen robes. By noon, the shade temperature (if you can find shade) may exceed 50°C. Underneath the robes, their bodies sweat, cooling themselves and the trapped microclimate. The heavy insulation protects the wearer from the extreme heat outside, and particularly from the direct and reflected radiant heat. There is no doubt that this traditional dress gives the wearer a considerable advantage (not least by encouraging stately movement), but of course it is not suitable for athletic activities!

In humid weather, sweat evaporates slowly, and thus cools less well. In response, the body produces even more sweat. If one wears just a suntan and a medallion, this may drip uselessly onto the ground instead of cooling, adding to the burden on the body's water resources. Clothing can absorb and evaporate sweat, creating a cool microclimate around the body, and can insulate against radiant heat. Although clothing may make one feel warmer and less comfortable, from the point of view of water economy and ultimate endurance, it is advantageous to wear something.

CHAPTER NINE

Drugs, hormones, and sundry potions — aids to performance?

Background

During the Seoul Olympics ten athletes were disqualified after testing positive for illegal drugs, and a number of others withdrew when it became clear that they could not avoid being tested. One of these was the Canadian sprinter, Ben Johnson, who lost his gold medal when anabolic steroids were found in his urine. As this is written, in May 1989, an investigation is taking place examining the use of drugs by Canadian athletes. At this stage it appears that, allegedly in the hope that clandestine drug use might improve athletics standards, Canadian officials may have turned a blind eye to drugs and hormones. They may even have warned athletes of future "random" drug tests. Some athletes additionally claim that they were encouraged to use drugs, and that they were told they had no chance of winning unless they did so. Meanwhile, some observers ironically suggest that the final cost of the investigation will be greater than the Canadian government's annual spending to promote athletics!

Ever since sports competition first began, athletes have looked for ways to improve their performance. In days of old, incantations were muttered, oracles consulted, and prayers directed to various gods. At the time of the original Olympics, dietary theories suggested that eating the flesh of a bull increased strength, while eating a lion's heart endowed one with courage. Closer to our own era, the secretion of the queen bee, "royal jelly", found favour. Today much, although not all, of this mythology has gone (diet books of little merit occasionally top the best-sellers charts). The methods used by sportsmen and women to boost performance can be grouped into four categories: diet, training, equipment, and drugs. The first three are time-honoured and accepted everywhere, while the fourth is officially and universally banned.

Unfortunately, there is no clear boundary between what is ac-

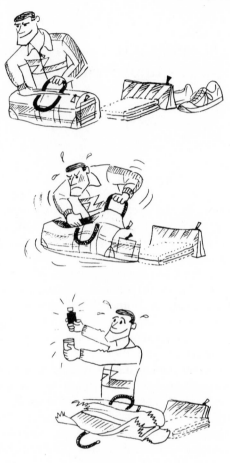

Fig. 9.1

ceptable and what is not. Thus, a professional athlete has no limitation on training, and his/her equipment may be supplied by a manufacturer. In contrast an amateur must train during spare time while earning a living and buy his/her own equipment. Competition between amateurs and professionals was thus felt to be unfair, and professionals were barred from the Olympics. This highlights a dilemma. Clearly, it is acceptable to spend a great deal of money on training and equipment, provided this comes from a

194

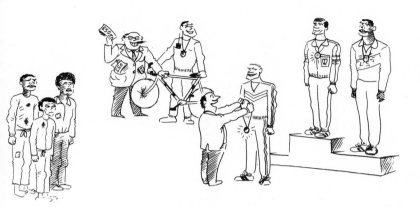

Fig. 9.2

sympathetic parent or employer but not from the public exhibition of one's skill — a curious form of logic.

Today, creative accounting combined with a more relaxed attitude make it hard to distinguish between the amateur and the professional. Professional tennis and football players are invited to the Olympics to compete against amateurs, and many track and field athletes draw "expenses" from trust funds provided by sponsors and advertisers, while others receive support from their governments. This has provided us with spectacular performers, but may have made it more difficult for young men and women from poor countries without access to equipment, coaching or sponsorship, to attain world ranking. Thus, several of today's top male sprinters are natives of the Caribbean, but run for other countries where they are able to obtain the facilities and support needed to succeed.

There is little doubt that certain drugs and hormones improve performance. If these were used under good medical supervision, many would also be safe. Some are used routinely for the treatment of disease. However, organisations such as the International Olympic Committee, the International Amateur Athletic Federation, and the American College of Sports Medicine have banned almost all pharmacological substances, thereby driving users underground, and legitimate doctors away.

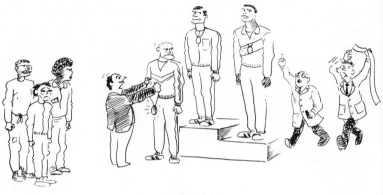

Fig. 9.3

People taking certain drugs for genuine ailments have been accused of trying to boost performance, while others may pretend to be ill as a cover for using a drug they believe will help them. Thus ephedrine, which might be taken for allergy or influenza and is found in nasal decongestants, is banned. Codeine, found in some headache tablets and cough syrups, is also banned.

The beta-blockers, used to steady limbs in competitive shooting or snooker, are a group of drugs used for hypertension. They are allowed if the sportsman is genuinely hypertensive. But is it fair to allow one competitor but not others to use this drug, particularly when the degree of hypertension which merits treatment varies widely among physicians?

Drugs and hormones are often self-administered or taken on the advice of a sports coach who lacks the skill to assess the dangers involved, or to notice untoward symptoms. During the current Canadian investigation into the use of drugs by sportsmen (above) one coach admitted he had no idea that anabolic steroids could be dangerous. The use of chemical agents to improve performance has become widespread, as is the certainty that many will cause harm.

Testing for drugs

Tests have been developed to detect many of the preparations which might be used by sportsmen. In the past these were chemi-

196

cal assays which depended on a separate laboratory procedure for each substance tested. The need to carry out a battery of tests for every substance made this slow, difficult, and expensive. Few tests could be completed and, for any particular athlete, the likelihood of detection was low. Today, most drugs and hormones can be detected using gas chromatography, or high pressure liquid chromatography.

This procedure depends on the speed with which the components of a sample move within a stationary medium which selectively absorbs and slows the passage of certain molecules, separating substances from each other. A sample of urine, suitably treated, is injected into the apparatus. Its vapour then moves through the chromatograpy column or tube. Various molecules are detected coming out of the apparatus at different times after injection, depending on the characteristics of the column, its contents, the solvent used, and the substances present in the sample. Sometimes a series of chemicals is injected into the apparatus after the sample to elute or "chase" certain molecules out of the column. The apparatus is calibrated by injecting chosen standards — small amounts of pure material — into it and noting the speed with which they pass through. These standards are selected from the substances one expects to find in the samples to be analysed.

Although chromatography equipment is expensive, tiny amounts of a wide range of substances can be detected at one time. A large number of samples can be assayed using it (the apparatus can run automatically). Most important, it is not necessary to know precisely which substances are being sought. The chromatograph can be calibrated after the samples are run, using standards of substances which one suspects may have been detected. This makes universal testing a possibility.

The results of such tests cannot be conclusive because chromatography does not positively identify a molecule. It simply shows that a specimen contains something which behaves like a particular substance. If anything suspicious is found, conventional chemical assays may be used to confirm the finding.

So-called "masking drugs" are used to make the detection of banned agents impossible. These work by passing through the chromatography apparatus at the same speed as the performance enhancing drug or hormone the sportsman is using. The masking drug appears at the detector at the same time as the drug, making it impossible to actually "see". Masking agents are substances neither normally present in the urine or blood, nor in legitimately used medicines. If found in the body, they can be assumed to be covering up something.

A masking agent prevents positive identification of a banned substance, but only by the methods of chromatography. The use of more conventional assay techniques would have little trouble "unmasking" the offender, but the labour and skill required to carry out these tests often prevents this from being done. Finding a masking agent could be sufficient to disqualify a competitor, but the rules of many sporting bodies would have to be changed to allow this.

Testing isn't straightforward

One problem with testing is that athletes often take a particular drug or hormone for several months, stopping well before a meet at which testing is likely. Some national athletics organisations have been accused of warning their athletes of future testing, giving them time to eliminate the substance and test "clean". If drug taking is to be discouraged, there must be random testing throughout the year. Recently, there was an interesting case of an athlete who had stopped taking drugs well before being tested, but still failed the test. He had removed and stored a quantity of his own blood several weeks before competition. This was infused back into his bloodstream on the eve of the meet (see blood doping, p. 99). Although the illegal substance had been eliminated from his body, it was well preserved in the stored blood, and he was disqualified!

To avoid detection, natural hormones such as testosterone have been used in place of synthetics (which might be cheaper and better). Of course, it is not possible to distinguish between the body's normal production of a hormone, and the same hormone administered by mouth or syringe. Officials must judge whether the amount of a hormone found in the urine or blood is too great to have been secreted naturally, and had to be administered by syringe or capsule.

To make things even more difficult, some of the drugs used by sportsmen are found in off-the-shelf items such as cough syrup, common cold medications, or headache tablets. It is hard to say with any certainty whether a substance has been taken innocently or deliberately.

Finally, trackside tests measure the concentration of a substance in an athlete's urine. This concentration depends on the rate at which urine is being formed. Suppose the athlete has just completed an endurance event and has lost a lot of sweat. The rate of urine formation will be low and anything it contains will be highly concentrated. On the other hand, an athlete participating in a sprint event will produce a more dilute urine which will contain far less of any drug. Yet another way to foil drug detection in urine is to "transplant" drug-free urine from a "clean" donor (often donated by the coach who recommended drug use) by catheter into the athlete's bladder! Neither method can be trusted to beat the sensitivity of today's sensitive tests. In any case, a drug test based on a blood sample is considerably more trustworthy, and its interpretation is more straightforward.

Drugs and hormones used by athletes

There are various types of preparations which are used to enhance performance. In general, these fall into five categories: stimulants, analgesics and anti-inflammatory agents, anabolic agents, anti-anxiety agents and diuretics.

stimulants

The stimulants include agents such as ephedrine, amphetamines and caffeine. They are used by cyclists, runners, footballers, and others who feel that these drugs will improve endurance or sharpen their reflexes. Another drug which belongs in this category is cocaine.

(a) *ephedrine and amphetamines*

These drugs wake up sleepy drivers. Although in drowsy people they give a sensation of alertness, there is no evidence that reflex movements in wide awake athletes or sportsmen are in any way speeded up or improved.

Ephedrine and amphetamines increase both blood pressure and heart rate, and relax bronchial muscles. These effects may be capable of increasing the rate at which blood circulates and of easing breathing somewhat. However, these tasks are nor-

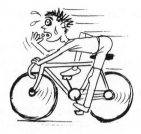 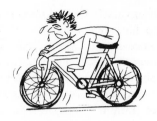

Fig. 9.4

mally accomplished by the body's own adrenaline and nor-adrenaline, and it is doubtful if amphetamines can actually improve on the natural effect. Tests show that neither speed nor power are improved. However, there is evidence of some gain in swimming, running and cycling endurance. This may well be due to a reduction in the perception of discomfort or fatigue.

The nature of this improvement is interesting. Many research workers have been unable to find a "statistically significant" change in performance due to these drugs. Even those who did obtain positive results admitted that these were small — in the range of 1–2%. Changes of this magnitude are rarely large enough to show up in scientifically conducted trials. However, it is by just such small margins that athletic competitions are won, and lost. Thus, even a very small improvement resulting from the use of amphetamine could make the difference between fame and oblivion! In the end, these drugs probably continue to be used more because their mood altering properties appeal to the athlete than because of any real benefit to performance.

Amphetamines also act as appetite suppressants and may be used by jockeys, boxers and wrestlers who wish to meet a target weight in order to compete in their chosen class. However, if a competitor has enough will power to adhere to a tough training schedule, finding a little more to maintain weight should be relatively simple.

Amphetamines are not without side effects, all of which are undesirable in an athlete. Among these are headaches, dizziness, confusion, and lack of judgement. Habituation to these drugs also occurs so that progressively larger doses are required to have an effect. Continued use may lead to dependence. Since amphetamines prevent sleep, barbiturates ("downers") may be taken to promote drowsiness, followed by more amphetamine ("uppers") later to wake up.

Any drug which reduces the sensation of pain, discomfort or fatigue is potentially dangerous because it suppresses mechanisms which protect against damage caused by over-exertion. There have been several cases where the deaths of professional cyclists through overheating were linked to the use of amphetamines.

In summary, it is important to note that although some research suggests that amphetamines may increase endurance, this effect is small and other work indicates that they have no effect. Also, speed and power are not affected. The disadvantages associated with their use, plus the fact that they are strictly banned, should be reason enough for these drugs never to be used by athletes.

(b) *caffeine*

Caffeine is found in coffee, tea, chocolate (which also contains a related substance, theobromine), headache tablets, cough medicines, and some carbonated beverages. Because these foods and products are widely available and consumed by most people, their use by athletes is difficult to control. Competition regulations simply limit the amount of caffeine which the urine may contain.

Caffeine has aroused interest recently because laboratory evidence has suggested that quite large doses (0.5 grams or 5–

Table 9.1 *Caffeine contents of some beverages and tablets (mg)*

Roasted coffee (cup)	60–150	
Instant coffee (cup)	40–100	
Decaffeinated	2–4	
Tea (cup)	20–70	
Cocoa (cup)	5	(+250 mg Theobromine)
Cola beverage (10 oz)	40–50	
Various analgesics and cold remedies	10–50	

8 cups of coffee or tea) may affect metabolism. In particular, it is claimed that caffeine promotes the use of fatty acids, sparing glycogen and improving endurance. Several experiments have shown that caffeine increases the rate at which fat stores are broken down and delivered to the circulation in a form which muscles can use. Adrenaline release is the main stimulus to fat mobilisation. Caffeine seems to potentiate its effectiveness in mobilising fat from stores. However, the effects of caffeine are notoriously variable and doses of over 600 mg per day may cause depression and other negative effects.

In laboratory tests using cycle ergometers one group of researchers has consistently found improved endurance, reduced muscle glycogen depletion, and even slightly increased work output. On the other hand, others fail to see any such improvement. Actual track tests have also yielded contradictory results.

It is worth examining possible reasons for this variability. The question is whether endurance performance is limited by (i) the rate at which fuels (fats, glucose, etc.) can be delivered to the working muscles, or whether the limitation is in (ii) the ability of muscle to oxidise the available fuel. If (i) is true, caffeine should increase endurance performance. If (ii) is true, there should be no effect. The limitation on an individual athlete's performance may be due to either factor.

Another property of caffeine is that it is a diuretic, increasing the rate of urine production, and causing water loss. By decreasing water reserves it may actually reduce endurance, particularly at high temperatures. The diuretic effect of caffeine may partly explain the unreliability of its reputed endurance promoting action.

In view of the variability of caffeine's action, and the high dose required to achieve even this variable effect, there is unlikely to be any benefit from a dose which would pass drug tests.

(c) *cocaine*

In its native Andes, cocaine is obtained by chewing the leaves of the coca bush. The slow absorption of relatively small amounts of cocaine taken in this form gives rise to far less addiction than does the rapid absorption of larger doses of the pure substance as taken in developed countries. Native

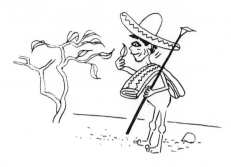

Fig. 9.5

Peruvians use coca leaves to suppress hunger when they are short of food, and to increase endurance during manual labour. It is this latter action which has attracted the attention of athletes.

Cocaine is readily absorbed by the intestine or by mucuous membranes (nose, mouth, etc.). Cocaine is fairly short-lived in the body, and half of a dose will be eliminated within one hour of ingestion. The effects of cocaine are very similar to those of amphetamine.

The drug is taken mainly for its effect on the brain, which it stimulates giving a sense of euphoria, strength and well-being. In terminal illness morphine may be given to alleviate pain, and cocaine is used to counter the morphine-induced depression. Co-ordination is apparently little affected by small doses of cocaine, but tremor, convulsions and vomiting occur after larger doses. As cocaine is eliminated from the body, depression follows euphoria. The extreme nature of this depression and the potent memory of the preceding pleasurable sensation are responsible for the drug's addictive properties.

Cocaine's effects on endurance are similar to those of amphetamine. By reducing the sensation of pain and fatigue, an individual is able to carry on longer. The ability to ignore pain and fatigue are short-term advantages. In the long term, this is likely to lead to damage and disability. It is also worth noting that many athletes who use neither cocaine nor amphetamine achieve much the same result through will power.

Cocaine increases the sensitivity of the cardiovascular system to stimulation by noradrenalin. This raises the heart rate and blood pressure, and tends to reduce blood flow to the limbs, adversely affecting the ability to lose heat. More alarmingly, the deaths of several athletes during competition appear to have been caused by obstruction of the coronary blood vessels in the heart, and linked to the use of cocaine.

This drug is illegal everywhere, extremely addictive, and dangerous. It should never be used.

diuretics

Since fighters (boxers, wrestlers, etc.) are put into weight classes, they can maximise their chances of winning by competing near the top of their weight range. They sometimes misjudge and are too heavy at the pre-match weigh-in. The rules give them a few hours in which to "make weight". This may be spent in a work-out session, often wearing a waterproof suit to promote sweating, which may dehydrate them by over two litres per hour. Unfortunately, such a work-out is fatiguing, and may reduce both endurance and performance in a subsequent match.

Diuretics are also used by such athletes, and by jockeys as an aid to weight loss. These drugs can force the kidney to produce over one litre of urine (1 kg) per hour, and without the fatigue of a work-out session. Diuretics are also dehydrating, and adversely affect work output. Occasionally, drugs which induce vomiting or diarrhoea might be used to shed weight.

Although the athlete often has time to drink water between the weigh-in and the competition, rehydration is rarely complete in

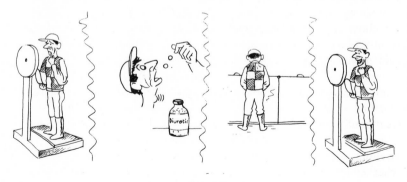

Fig. 9.6

such a short time. After dehydration, it often takes 24 hours or longer to properly restore body fluids to their normal volume.

None of these rapid weight loss techniques should ever be used. However induced, dehydration lowers endurance and peak work output. If an endurance or middle distance activity is undertaken, dehydration increases the likelihood of thermal injury — collapse due to a combination of overheating and circulatory failure (see p. 182). The effects of such a collapse can be serious.

Athletes may also use diuretics to mask their use of drugs. By greatly increasing the flow of urine, diuretics dilute any drug or its breakdown products, making it more difficult to detect. This use of diuretics, after an athletic event, is probably harmless. However, modern biochemical tests are so sensitive that such a crude attempt to avoid detection is probably futile. During the 1988 Seoul Olympics, several weight lifters used catheters to fill their bladders with drug-free or "clean" urine (referred to as a "urine transplant"), donated by colleagues, in order to dilute the anabolic steroids present. Even this apparently foolproof plan failed and they were disqualified.

analgesics and anti-inflammatory agents

Analgesics and anti-inflamatory agents cover a range of substances from aspirin to hydrocortisone. Analgesics relieve the pain of injury, while anti-inflammatory drugs relieve swelling and the associated discomfort. None of these substances has any effect on performance in the healthy individual and, opiates (pethidine, heroin, opium, etc.) apart, their use in competitive sport is not prohibited.

Since analgesics reduce pain, it has been thought that they may somehow "cure" muscle damage caused by overwork (see p. 242). A number of studies have shown neither visible nor chemical evidence of any reduction in the degree of damage, or in the speed of recovery. Even their pain-reducing action is in some doubt. In double blind trials where neither subject nor scientist knew whether a drug or a placebo was being administered, the two treatments had similar effects on the degree of pain reported.

Anti-inflammatory drugs and hormones relieve and reduce the swelling and redness associated with injury. Damage to a tissue, whether by infection or by physical injury, releases various substances such as intracellular proteins, enzymes, histamine, prostaglandins, etc. Some of these render capillaries leaky so that fluid leaves the circulation, causing local oedema or swelling. This fluid is accompanied by white cells which devour damaged tissue, and remove it from the site. Protein leakage increases the osmotic pressure of the interstitial fluid (p. 174) so that the oedema fluid cannot be readily reabsorbed into the plasma. Eventually the leaked protein is returned to the blood by the lymphatic system, along with the white cells plus any cellular debris they have "eaten", and the swelling subsides.

Aspirin (and similar non-steroidal drugs) act as anti-inflammatory agents by blocking the formation of prostaglandins. However, there are many mediators of inflammation so that the non-steroidals are not particularly effective in halting it following injury. For that the corticosteroid hormones and their analogues must be used.

The glucocorticoids have several anti-inflammatory properties: (1) They inhibit the manufacture of protein everywhere but in the liver. This includes the lymphatic tissue where white cells are made. (2) They are very effective antihistamines, preventing its release and the fluid leakage it causes. (3) They block the action of some of the enzymes released by damaged tissue, which participate in the inflammation process. However, the inflammatory process is the means by which the body's repair systems move into a damaged tissue to start healing. Thus suppression of inflammation slows healing. Also, the inhibition of protein synthesis caused by these hormones is another unwelcome action. This slows the manufacture of new tissue and retards healing. For these reasons, the dose of anti-inflammatory steroids must be kept low, and as brief as possible.

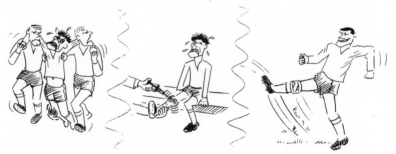

Fig. 9.7 Anti-inflammatory steroids such as hydrocortisone may be injected directly into a swollen joint to relieve pain.

One aspect of the use of the anti-inflammatory steroids may be beneficial. Although one effect of inflammation is to increase local blood flow (note the warmth of an injured site), severe swelling increases local pressure which can reduce the flow of blood to the site of injury and slow healing. Reducing severe swelling allows more blood to reach the site of injury.

If administered to the whole body, anti-inflammatory steroids would promote the breakdown of muscle protein and weaken muscle, an unwelcome effect! For this reason, they are usually injected directly into an injured joint, so that little escapes into the circulation.

The problem arises from the use to which these drugs are put. They are often administered to athletes who have injured themselves in training or in competition, and who wish to carry on. Pain is a sign to the body indicating that something is wrong. The use of drugs which suppress pain is likely to lead to further and more severe injury.

anabolic agents
(a) steroids

Anabolic steroids came into prominence recently due to publicity generated following the 1988 Seoul Olympics. Several competitors were found to have used these substances, and others withdrew from competition when it became clear that they could not escape testing. Canadian athletics is now experiencing a cathartic inquiry into the use of drugs. Various Canadian athletes have testified that they obtained their supplies with the help of American athletes. Meanwhile the Americans are (unconvincingly) protesting their innocence. With the help of "Glasnost" the Russian news media reported that many of their sportsmen and women used steroids during training, stopping prior to the Olympics. Their national squad was (unofficially) tested for drugs just before competition to ensure that all members would pass any official test they might have to undergo.

What are anabolic steroids? There are over a dozen substances available which mimic the male hormone testosterone. These analogues of testosterone are also called androgenic steroids. Some can be taken orally while others must be injected intramuscularly.

Males produce considerably more testosterone than females. Testosterone is the hormone responsible for the generally greater muscle bulk and strength of males compared to females (anabolic properties). It is also responsible for the secondary sexual characteristics (androgenic properties), which include the male-pattern hair distribution and the tendency towards aggression displayed by many males. If strength training is undertaken, their high rate of testosterone production allows males to achieve greater gains in strength than females. In fact, "trainability" in both sexes peaks at around age 25, paralleling their testosterone production (Fig. 2.12, and p. 24).

If testosterone is responsible for the natural strength of males, then by administering this hormone, or synthetic substances similar to testosterone, it ought to be possible to make both males and females grow stronger. In fact, it is not that simple. In females, steroids always produce gains in strength which begin to approach the muscle development of males. In clinical medicine, testosterone and anabolic steroids have been used to restore muscle bulk in patients with muscle-wasting diseases — and they are effective.

In theory, if a little testosterone (the natural secretion) is good, then more (as synthetic anabolic steroids) ought to be better. Unfortunately, the response to testosterone saturates, so that it and other androgens are most effective in people with a low natural production. Thus, a low dose will have a

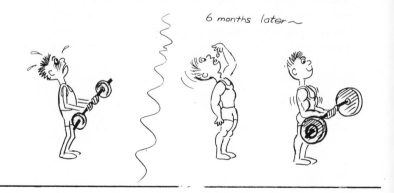

6 months later

Fig. 9.8

dramatic effect in a woman or in a testosterone deficient patient, while a normal male would require more than ten times the amount.

One problem is that when androgens are administered, the body's natural secretion of testosterone diminishes. A low rate of testosterone secretion persists for months after stopping anabolic steroids. In fact, sub-normal testosterone production is one way that the use of anabolic steroids (current or recent) may be deduced, despite the administration of so-called "masking drugs" (p. 197). Other clues are that the prolonged use of anabolic steroids alters the rate at which various other hormones are secreted, as well as some more visible effects.

The synthetic anabolic steroids were designed with the aim of emphasising the anabolic (muscle building) effect and minimising the androgenic (male sexual) properties which are characteristic of the natural hormone. However, it has not been possible to separate these effects.

In females, the use of anabolic steroid hormones has many undesirable actions including baldness, excessive hair growth on the body, infertility, plus the loss of subcutaneous fat and feminine shape. Indeed, the term "East German female athlete" conjures up an image of the square-rigged, muscular, and unlovely women who excelled at the shot-put some twenty years ago. These masculinising effects should have restricted the use of anabolic steroids to males. However, the recent Canadian enquiry into drugs in sport has revealed that a number of champion female sprinters took these substances over many years. We must assume that judicious restraint saved them from the most obvious side effects of these substances.

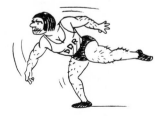

Fig. 9.9

The results of many experiments agree that anabolic steroids increase body weight. However, in carefully controlled trials the expected increase in strength has not always been seen. The failure of strength to develop may be due to inadequate or inappropriate training. Where greater strength is seen, this may simply be due to heightened aggression helping the athlete make a maximum effort. Also, experiments carried out under medical supervision must be ethical and cannot put the subject at risk. For this reason, the doses used in legitimate research have, of necessity, been conservative. Athletes playing the game of win-at-all-costs have cheerfully given themselves *OVER 100 TIMES* the recommended dose of anabolic steroids. It is not surprising that their coaches and quacks often administered the veterinary formulations (identical, but concentrated and in larger bottles) — and even then, the illstarred Canadian, Ben Johnson, was reportedly taking thirty times the dose recommended for horses!

There is a widespread belief that muscle or tendon damage heals faster in people taking anabolic steroids. Although these hormones do increase the rate at which tissues manufacture protein, professional opinion discounts this theory. Muscle development outstrips that of tendons, and larger, more powerful muscles are more likely to be damaged in use. The use of anabolic steroids is associated with an increased tendency of muscle and tendon damage in weight lifters. This is very likely caused by increased aggressiveness, driving them to lift greater weights and perhaps even to less careful technique.

It is worth noting here that muscle and joint injuries anyway heal more quickly in trained than in sedentary individuals. This is due to differences in vascularity. Athletes' muscles and bones have a greater number of capillaries, and the improved blood supply speeds healing. Anabolic steroids have no effect on blood flow, and cannot promote healing in this way. However, coupled with the rapid recovery of many athletes, this negative effect of steroid use is often missed.

Used in the young person, testosterone and its synthetic analogues stunt growth. Indeed, they may have been used to keep the stature of gymnasts small. They are suspected of causing osteoporosis (see p. 232) and leukaemia. These hormones cause infertility in both sexes, although permanent infertility is rare. However, the main danger of anabolic steroids is that they encourage the development of various types of liver disease. These include liver failure, cancer of the liver and a usually rare form of hepatitis (yellowed or jaundiced eyes may be seen as a result). The incidence of some types of liver disease in athletes is many times higher than expected, suggesting extensive steroid use.

Testosterone and the anabolic steroids used by athletes also tend to cause hypertension. Steroid-using athletes are more likely to be hypertensive than their un-drugged colleagues. Since many steroid-using athletes participate in sports like weight lifting, during which blood pressure rises spectacularly for short periods, hypertension may be particularly dangerous to them.

The use of anabolic steroids by trained athletes also causes a sharp drop in the amount of high density lipoprotein (one of the forms in which blood-borne cholesterol exists) in the blood, with the possibility that this may increase the risk of coronary heart disease. Minor symptoms of steroid use include acne, deepening of the voice, and increased facial hair. Many men using these hormones have developed gynaecomastia — enlarged breasts.

Anabolic steroids alter personality. Male athletes taking these drugs become more hostile, aggressive and violent ("steroid rage", or "roid rage"). This psychological change may be of considerable benefit in strength oriented sports. In certain competitive contact sports such as American football and ice hockey, aggression may be the specific effect sought.

Finally, anabolic steroids are addictive. This effect is different from the addiction to heroin or nicotine. Athletes are so convinced that the drugs are required to be competitive in their sport that they will not stop taking them, even when they are told that they are already suffering from serious side effects which may become dangerous!

If the use of anabolic steroids was confined to the small world of competitive athletics, the problem would be a minor one and manageable. However, teenagers involved in school sports are taking them as are members of body-building clubs and gyms. They are even being used casually by young men who simply wish to look good (and perhaps feel good) with-

H

out making the effort required to build muscles more conventionally. They all believe that anabolic steroids can perform body-building miracles, and there is no evidence for that.

Illegality has driven anabolic steroid use underground. Accordingly, it is neither possible to obtain reliable information about the long term effects of anabolic steroids, nor to estimate how many people use them. Opinion among athletes suggest that between 25% to 90% of competitive sportsmen have taken anabolic steroids at some time. The wide range reflects uncertainty because use of these substances by competitive athletes is illegal and because many sports bodies are now willing to ban athletes known to have used them.

(b) growth hormone — a substitute for anabolic steroids?

Growth hormone should have much the same effect on muscle growth as the anabolic steroids, minus their androgenic action. It increases the retention of amino acids and the synthesis of protein. Furthermore, it promotes fat mobilisation and metabolism.

Growth hormone is a protein, and most protein hormones from one species of animal tend to be inactive in other species. Growth hormone from pigs, sheep or cows is ineffective in man. Up to now, human growth hormone for clinical purposes has been obtained from cadavers, and is both rare and expensive. The very small quantities available to date have been used to treat children who are dwarfed or stunted because they are deficient in the hormone. Genetic engineering techniques will soon make the hormone more readily and cheaply available, and abuse by athletes is likely to become common. Indeed, the large amounts of money in track and field sports today has made it possible for some athletes to obtain this hormone, to the great disadvantage of some hormone-deficient child. Fortunately for these children, genetically engineered growth hormone is now being produced and will be licenced for use very soon.

When growth hormone does become widely available, the side-effects of its abuse will be gigantism (excessive growth, but in proportion) in youths and acromegaly (overgrowth and deformation of certain bones, particularly in the hands, feet and face) in adults. These bone changes are irreversible, and predispose the victim to arthritis. Growth hormone is also likely to cause enlargement of heart muscle by increasing the thickness of its individual muscle cells. This change increases the diffusion distance for oxygen (p. 18) and makes the heart more vulnerable to hypoxia (oxygen shortage).

The consequences of these side effects ought to deter potential users. However, the temptation of potential improvements in athletic prowess will be hard to resist, however serious the danger. Growth hormone has a half-life in the body of just 25 minutes, and is undetectable after just one day of abstinence. This should make the temptation to use it almost irresistible.

anti-anxiety agents

Anti-anxiety agents are used to calm people. This would be of great use to precision performers such as snooker players, archers, golfers, figure skaters, and marksmen. In all cases the potential for improved performance exists if muscle tremor can be eliminated or reduced. There are two classes of anti-anxiety agents: the tranquillizers (Reserpine, Valium, etc), and the anti-hypertensive β-blockers. Alcohol is also classed as an anti-anxiety drug.

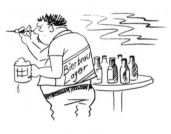

Fig. 9.10

The β-blockers were originally developed for lowering blood pressure in hypertensive patients, and may also be used to relieve the pain of angina. They act by preventing some of the actions of adrenalin and noradrenalin. Tranquillizers, which reduce the amounts of adrenalin and noradrenalin released within the body, are also used. In addition to calming anxiety, these drugs lower the heart's stroke volume (the amount of blood pumped at each stroke) and the heart rate. A large stroke volume can actually cause the body to move by enough to affect precision in these activities.

Marksmen (archery, shooting), snooker players, ski jumpers, bobsledders, figure skaters, gymnasts, sailors, divers, etc. may all derive an advantage from the use of such drugs. These are sports in which co-ordination is all important, while strength and endurance contribute little to success.

The biathlon is another sport where β-blockers may be used advantageously. This Winter Olympic event combines cross-country skiing and shooting, or speed and endurance with marksmanship. Immediately after the heavy exertion of skiing, the volume of blood pumped by the heart is large, making it particularly difficult to hold the rifle steady and aim accurately. The use of β-blockers improves precision, however, the potential effects on speed and endurance are no help to the competitor.

By lowering the stroke volume, these drugs reduce the maximum output of the heart, and are likely to limit aerobic performance. Various workers have looked at the effects of these drugs on VO_{2MAX}, but the results have been inconclusive. β-blockers also reduce the ability to use glycogen and to mobilise fats for metabolism, both of which have serious implications for endurance. It may be that, by careful choice of the actual drug used and its dose, these adverse effects might be avoided. However, by improving the flow of blood to the hearts of angina patients, β-blockers usually improve performance.

Like virtually all drugs, the use of β-blockers is banned in competition. However, if a competitor can show that the drugs have been perscribed as a treatment for hypertension, they may be allowed. The problem arises in defining hypertension. Since the β-blockers seem to improve accuracy, a surprising number of archers, shooters and snooker players turn out to be "hypertensive"!

Alcohol is an old standby. Its calming effect may assist in improving marksmanship with firearms, but is less likely to do so in archery where far more strength is required. The dose must be finely judged, since too much will make standing difficult, let alone any attempt at accuracy. Alcohol is banned by the governing bodies of some sports, but not by others.

"Magic" potions — various over-the-counter and legal substances

Sportsmen and women also use a number of aids to performance which truly must be labelled potions. Again, it is the quest for performance which drives them, and the knowledge that the margin separating the victor from the also-ran is exceedingly small. This means that even the placebo effect (if you think it is doing you good, then it probably is!) of a useless treatment may be important.

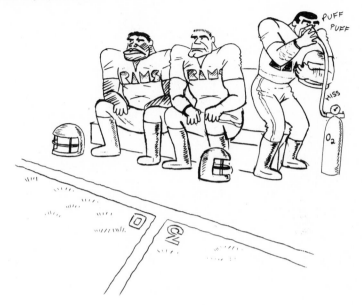

Fig. 9.11

oxygen breathing

Breathing a gas mixture enriched in oxygen has been shown to increase the VO_{2MAX}. Although the magnitude of this increase is no more than 5%, the closeness of some athletic contests is such that any improvement may be thought worthwhile and be eagerly sought. Thus, oxygen cylinders have been seen on the sidelines at professional American Football matches so that players can grab a quick whiff when they feel distressed.

If oxygen offers an athlete the promise of improved performance, what of the urban pedestrian? In Tokyo, coin-operated roadside machines vend a few gulps of oxygen to people oppressed by the heavy pollution in one of the world's most congested cities.

Oxygen breathing is quite useless. Its effects last no longer than it takes to blow it out of the lungs, or less than thirty seconds. Unless an athlete wears breathing gear continuously, no benefit can result. Very few activities would be unhindered by the weight and bulk of such equipment. Even in climbing expeditions at high altitude, where thin air severely hinders performance, many climbers are of the opinion that the use of an oxygen breathing apparatus slows them by more than it helps.

potassium and calcium

During and after hard exercise, potassium and calcium escape from the working muscles and appear in the blood. Some purveyors of health foods have suggested that oral replacement of these ions will improve performance.

This is quite untrue. While potassium is indeed lost from working muscle, the body's stores of this mineral are very large, and there is no need to take any additional material in the form of electrolyte drinks or tablets. Moreover, the quantities of potassium which might be taken in this way are small compared to the intake provided by a normal diet.

With respect to calcium, the situation is different. Normal muscle fibres (cells) lose very little or no calcium, however hard they work. If increased amounts of calcium do appear in the bloodstream following exercise, this indicates that muscle fibres have been damaged. Damaged cells lose part of their contents, and calcium is probably the least important of these.

In any case, calcium is so vital for the activation of many processes in living cells that it is a priority requirement. If, for any reason, it is in short supply, the body obtains its needed calcium by "mining" it from the vast reservoir in the skeleton (see p. 232). With respect to the activation of muscle contraction, there is never a shortage of calcium, so no improvement in speed or power can occur if additional calcium is taken in the diet.

A normal "western" diet provides considerably more calcium than a person requires. The only people who risk calcium deficiency are vegans, whose diets exclude not only meat, eggs, and fish, but dairy products as well. The diets of Asian countries, where dairy products are not consumed, also tend to be poor in calcium, although even there calcium deficiency is far from commonplace. It is worth noting that calcium deficiency does exist in people whose diets are very odd, particularly if they are also pregnant or lactating. Even in severe deficiency, there is always enough calcium to produce normal muscle activation.

sodium chloride (salt)

Sodium supplements, as pills or under the guise of electrolyte beverages, have been used by athletes participating in endurance events for some time. Although a great deal of salt may be lost in sweat following exertion at high temperatures, in general, salt or sodium supplements are probably not useful.

During an endurance event, fluids are not well absorbed from the intestine because its blood supply is greatly reduced, as is its general level of activity. The addition of salt to the ingested fluid slows absorption even more. This ensures that, in general, useful quantities of salt cannot be consumed while the subject is active.

Of greater importance is the effect of high salt intake on the body's sodium conservation mechanisms. If the body is allowed to run short of salt, it secretes a hormone, aldosterone, which limits the loss of salt in the sweat. Salt supplements suppress aldosterone production and prevent normal salt conservation. Thus, the habitual use of salt supplements ensures that large amounts of salt will be lost whenever sweat production is high, and this loss requires replacement. In this sense, salt supplementation is "addictive".

A frequently observed consequence of endurance athletics in hot climates is heat stroke and collapse. This is due to the loss of large amounts of fluid from the body, and is readily treated by giving salt and water (and, of course, cooling the victim). However, if salt supplements are avoided during training, endurance and performance in the heat are improved (see p. 186).

sodium bicarbonate (baking soda)

During brief, intense activity, large quantities of lactic acid are produced by muscles engaged in anaerobic metabolism. This acidifies the blood (lowers the pH) and makes it more difficult for muscle to transfer its surplus lactic acid to the blood. Accumulation of lactic acid contributes to the onset of fatigue in sprint activity. It is logical to expect that any improvement in the ability to neutralise lactic acid should improve anaerobic endurance.

Observations made on people living and working at high altitudes in the Andes contradict this. Their high altitude habitat causes them to ventilate their lungs more vigorously than a sea level dweller. This makes them lose a great deal of carbon dioxide, and they must compensate by reducing their blood content of bicarbonate. Work tests have shown that these people perform perfectly well in anaerobic sprint activity, apparently suffering very little disadvantage from their bicarbonate deficit. However, workers and peasants in the Andes are not in competition, and remain blissfully unconcerned if trudging home after work takes them a little longer than it might.

The ingestion of some twenty grams of sodium bicarbonate (baking soda) a few hours before sprint activity renders the blood mildly alkaline and increases its capacity to accept and neutralise acid. In theory therefore, the body ought to be able to cope with more lactic acid.

The results of a number of tests were inconclusive, with some individuals exhibiting better speed and short term endurance, while others failed to show any change. However, none performed less well.

Sodium bicarbonate is considered to be non-toxic. Because it is available, cheap, and used orally, banning cannot realistically be policed. Moreover, since it either has no effect or improves performance, its use is a one-way bet — the athlete can't lose!

The temptation is to argue that if a little is good, more might be better. In large enough quantities, even sodium bicarbonate may become toxic. Fortunately, unmistakable warnings in the form of vomiting and diarrhoea are likely to prevent any really serious consequences.

amino acids
Sports and fitness publications are full of advertisements for countless amino acid supplements. These make many claims, including the suggestion that a particular combination of amino acids can be rapidly absorbed and incorporated into muscle, resulting in larger, stronger muscles.

These claims are without foundation. Although the lack of protein or of a specific amino acid could be the cause of poor muscle development, most people living in the "western" world have a diet which is adequately rich in protein. Under such conditions, any additional protein ingested will simply be burnt for energy or converted into glycogen and stored.

It has been suggested that body-builders do not consume enough protein to build muscle as fast as they would like. This is likely to be true only if the individual was also taking anabolic steroids or growth hormone which stimulate the rapid manufacture of protein in muscle. Potential customers for these products living in underdeveloped countries are unlikely to be able to afford them.

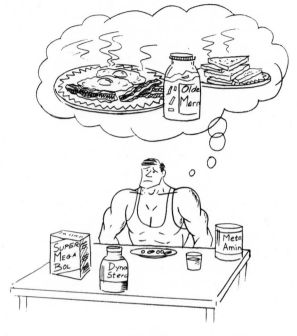

Fig. 9.12

In any case, they can achieve the same effects more cheaply by adding an egg or two to whatever diet they usually eat.

In any case, simply eating random amino acids will not help build protein, even in people whose diet is deficient. In order to be incorporated into protein, amino acids must be taken in the correct proportions, and eaten at a single sitting because the body is unable to store them for more than a few hours.

Endorphins

Endorphins do not really belong in a chapter on drugs and potions because they are not administered or taken voluntarily. Moreover, they certainly cannot be grouped with "potions". The term endorphin refers to a group of opium-like substances which are produced and released within the brain. They have analgesic and calming effects similar to those produced by opium and morphine, and this similarity is strengthened by the observation that their effects are antagonised by the same drugs which block the effects of opiates.

The endorphins are only released under conditions of stress, which can be emotional, brought about by prolonged strenuous exercise, or by chronic pain. Endorphin release can also be stimulated by acupuncture. It is thought that the analgesic effects ascribed to acupuncture treatment are mediated by the release of endorphins.

The release of endorphins as a consequence of endurance exercise is thought to be the cause of the "runner's high" — thirty years ago this was called a "runner's calm" or "second wind". This state of mind appears after more than twenty minutes of endurance activity, and can last for several hours.

Interestingly, this prolonged calm is followed by a sensation of agitation two or three days after the bout of exercise — promptly relieved by more exercise! Several people have suggested that endurance exercise (particularly marathon running) may produce a state of dependency or mild addiction which is the consequence of endorphin secretion.

One characteristic of opiate dependency is a progressive increase in the dose required to make the addict feel "normal". Again, it has been said that joggers tend to steadily increase the distance they run in a manner reminiscent of addiction. It may not be. As joggers run, they become more fit, and need to go progressively faster and farther to experience the same level of stress — and therefore to "dose" themselves with the same quantity of endor-

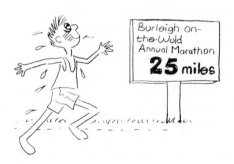

Fig. 9.13

phins. The manner in which endorphins are released (only after severe and prolonged stress) seems calculated to minimise the likelihood of dependency.

The "purpose" of the endorphins may be to relieve the pain and discomfort of endurance exercise. Pain is certainly suppressed during exercise and injury may occur entirely un-noticed, only to be discovered afterwards. The endorphins also appear to play a role in regulating the release of other hormones during periods of stress. There is some evidence that endorphin release may play a role in causing the infertility experienced by peasant women during times of hard work and food shortage, and in female endurance athletes (see p. 236).

It has recently been suggested that endorphins may be a factor in collapse during fun runs. Plasma endorphin concentrations were twice as high in a group of runners who collapsed towards the end of a half-marathon than in another group of runners who did not collapse. The high endorphin concentration may have prevented the collapsed runners from sensing their growing distress and responding to it by stopping. Clearly, the same reasoning can be applied to the use of amphetamine, cocaine, or even caffeine to improve endurance, and probably to increase the risk of collapse.

Conclusion

Even if drugs and potions often appear not to improve performance, the fact that they are believed to do so will ensure their continued use despite any official ban. Eventually, the use of certain drugs by sportsmen may well be sanctioned — just as professionalism has now been accepted in many sports. In principle, the use of drugs and hormones differs little from access to good coaching, nutritional advice, or the use of the best equipment.

Perhaps what really should be questioned is modern attitudes. The old Olympic ideal — that taking part is more important than winning — has been turned on its head. This is complemented by the attitude of the modern spectator who now seems more interested in watching perfection than in supporting a sportsman or a team which truly represents his locality.

In the end, the quest for ultimate performance is the problem. It is the athletes' equivalent of an arms race to which there can be no limit. Athletes are already dying, directly or indirectly, because of

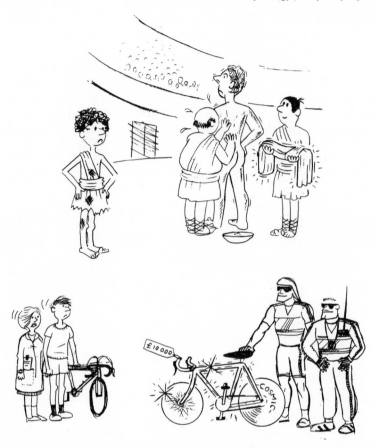

Fig. 9.14 Competition has always been unfair.

excessive drug taking. Curiously, banning is not particularly helpful because this ensures that the use of drugs is not supervised by
qualified medical personnel, and is thus more dangerous than it
need be.

CHAPTER TEN

Is exercise good for you?

Athletes have a "healthy" image. Athletic activities and training often take place outdoors and the participants tend to be tanned, and "glow" somewhat. They are often lean, or if large, tend to be well muscled rather than fat. The appearance of any active person is the opposite of our mental image of illness. Not long ago, pictures of sporty-looking people engaged in outdoor activities were used to advertise cigarettes. This powerful image was so successful that this type of advertising was banned when the tide of medical opinion finally turned against smoking. Today, similar pictures are still used to sell cars, clothing, carbonated beverages, fast food, and other products which have little to do with physical fitness or sports.

The media have pushed the view that regular exercise is good for you and that it is synonymous with health. Governments are promoting sports and physical activity as "healthy". The U.K.

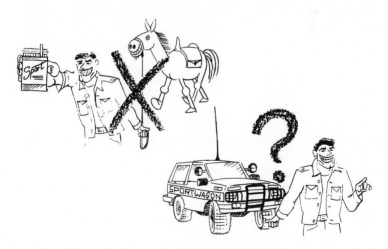

Fig. 10.1 *The concepts of sport and activity are often used to advertise products having nothing to do with either.*

223

slogan is "Sport for All", while Canada's is "Participaction". Manufacturers of sports equipment and clothing have also capitalised on the health image of exercise. Publicity has reinforced the association between health and exercise, but it is true?

What does "good for you" mean?

Before answering this question, the type of exercise, its intensity, frequency, and duration must be defined. There is a world of difference between two hours of golf, one hour of fast squash, or fifteen minutes of "pumping iron". Only after specifying the activity can one argue about the benefits which might arise.

The concept of "benefit" also must be defined. Are we hoping that exercise might reduce the likelihood of certain kinds of disease, partially reverse some adverse symptoms, or perhaps even increase our lifespan? Alternatively, benefit might be defined as an improved "quality of life" — whatever that might be!

Consider two broad classes of exercise: strength training or "isometric" exercise; and endurance training or "isotonic" exercise.

strength training

Weight lifting, working on certain gymnasium apparatus, or isometric effort based on straining against an immovable object, develop muscular strength and increase muscle size. The effects of such training are largely limited to improvements in muscle power. However, this power can be used only for short periods of time. In addition, the effects of strength training are concentrated on the specific muscles which were used during training, and even to the particular movements undertaken. To achieve a balanced result, a wide variety of training activities must be carried out.

To increase strength, it is necessary to load muscles heavily. The load applied is usually over 70% of a muscle's maximum tension. Clearly, the more often such a load is applied, the greater the training effect. However, work carried out with such heavy loads is rapidly fatiguing, and cannot be long sustained. Because of its necessarily short duration, weight lifting has a relatively small effect on oxygen consumption. Therefore, little stress is applied to either the metabolic systems which supply the energy for work or to the cardiovascular system which delivers it, and both respond poorly to this form of training.

224

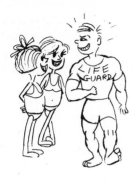

Fig. 10.2

It might be argued that the main benefit of strength training is cosmetic. The altered body shape, plus increased muscle size and definition are considered attractive and desirable in their own right. The only other identifiable benefit of pure strength training is improved resistance to overload injury. Thus, a body builder is less likely to strain his or her back when digging in the garden or lifting a heavy load, than an untrained person.

A minor negative effect of strength training is that the body's extra weight of muscle is permanently carried around, whatever the activity. This places an extra strain on the cardiovascular system. However, the owner of a well muscled, powerful body is unlikely to complain of this, or even to notice.

It is worth pointing out that relatively few people undertake pure strength training. Weight lifters and body builders generally include some jogging and circuit training in their programme, thus achieving a mixture of strength and endurance, but usually biassed towards the former.

endurance training
Endurance training is achieved by working regularly at relatively light work loads. Just two weeks of twenty minutes of daily activity vigorous enough to raise the pulse rate to 160 beats per minute can achieve a clear improvement in performance. However, the effectiveness of such a modest training regime depends on the initial level of physical fitness. Subjects who were fairly fit to begin with would see little change, while more sedentary subjects are likely to experience an encouraging improvement in both endurance and speed.

The effects of endurance training on muscle strength are small. Muscle strength is marginally increased by light, regular use, however heavy loading is needed to achieve a clear improvement. Instead, by regularly increasing the demand for oxygen, fuel and heat dissipation, endurance training improves the performance of the body's accessory systems — the cardiovascular, respiratory and thermoregulatory systems, and particularly the metabolic performance of the whole body. How might these changes be beneficial to health, disease resistance, or longevity?

This chapter considers the effects of endurance exercise on a few medical conditions: cardiovascular disease, obesity, and osteoporosis. Two problems arising from vigorous exercise, heat exhaustion and muscle damage, are also discussed.

Cardiovascular disease

Cardiovascular disease falls into three broad categories. Dramatic and very worrying are coronary heart disease, or "heart attack" and angina pectoris (severe chest pain on exercise). Stroke, or sudden damage to parts of the brain, is another form of cardiovascular disease common in industrial countries. Stroke is closely linked to high blood pressure or hypertension, a third member of this group.

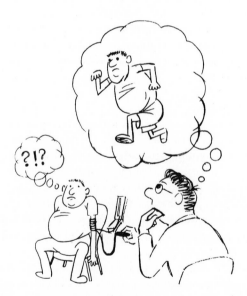

Fig. 10.3 There is a widespread belief that cardiovascular disease can be prevented by energetic regular activity.

Coronary heart disease and exercise

what is coronary heart disease?

Coronary heart disease is caused by a narrowing of the arteries which supply the heart muscle, the coronary arteries. This partial obstruction is due to deposits of cholesterol and clotted blood on the vessel wall, reducing blood flow. The severe pain of angina occurs whenever the heart muscle requires more oxygen than the partly blocked blood vessels can supply. Angina may also be caused by a spasm of the smooth muscle within the coronary arteries suddenly, but temporarily, reducing the heart's blood supply. Heart attacks are probably caused by blood clots dislodged from a coronary artery. These travel down the artery until they lodge in a smaller branch, plugging it. The sudden reduction in oxygen supply to a part of the heart muscle usually causes permanent damage. If the damaged area is large, the mass of heart muscle remaining may not be strong enough to continue supplying an adequate blood flow to the body, and death occurs.

what has lifestyle to do with it?

A number of doctors working in Africa and Asia suggested fifty years ago that lifestyle could affect the incidence of cardiovascular disease. They noticed that patients with heart attacks or angina were seldom seen, and on autopsy atherosclerosis was rare. As recently as 1982, at a clinical scientific meeting in Zimbabwe a rural doctor reported a case of angina in a middle aged peasant woman and asked whether anybody else in the audience had seen a similar case! Meanwhile, coronary heart disease became a major killer in Europe and America — particularly as antibiotics and other drugs had greatly reduced the risk of death from other causes.

Of course, it is unrealistic to compare peasants from the third world to the urban population of industrial countries. It is maybe invalid even to compare industrial populations whose social structures differ. Thus differences in lifestyle, diet, environment and genes make a meaningful comparison between Italians, Germans and Finns difficult, while realistic comparisons between urban Japanese and their American counterparts are probably impossible.

A few studies have looked at the long term effects of exercise. In some experiments volunteers participated in exercise programmes over a number of years. Various measurements were made at the start, and repeated again after years of activity. These studies were plagued with dropouts, often ending with only one quarter of the original volunteers still active. Risk factors associated with coronary heart disease (including plasma cholesterol, obesity, and blood pressure) were studied. The researchers were unable to show that long term physical activity is associated with a reduction in these risk factors.

Surveys collect data from large groups of people. Comparisons can be made between people who exercise regularly and those who are sedentary. With very large numbers, one may count how many individuals suffer from cardiovascular disease over the years. Such surveys show that exercise is associated with a reduction in coronary heart disease. However, surveys can be criticised. People with angina or breathlessness carry a high risk of coronary heart disease. The pain and discomfort they suffer when active ensures that they remain sedentary, removing themselves and their high risk from the exercise group. Another difficulty with surveys is that people who exercise tend to differ from more sedentary folk. They often eat "healthy" diets, avoid smoking, and are slim. These differences all reduce the risk of coronary heart disease, making the interpretation of survey results difficult.

On the other hand, animal experiments have shown how exercise might protect against coronary heart disease. The hearts of exercising animals become more vascular so that the diameter and number of coronary arteries increases. When atherosclerosis does occur, the greater number of small arteries ensures that, if one branch does become blocked, nearby parallel vessels may be able to supply blood to the affected region, reducing the severity of a heart attack. In addition, the increased diameter of the coronary arteries renders them less susceptible to blockage.

Exercise is used as therapy for survivors of heart attacks. This involves putting heart patients on an exercise programme of gradually increasing work intensity. Most of the participants in such a programme are restored to normal activity levels within six months, and half eventually become more physically fit than they had been before their heart attack.

The topic of exercise and coronary heart disease has generated a lot of research. Some is poor and only causes controversy. What is not controversial is that endurance athletes of all ages, including

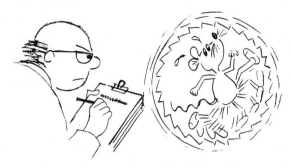

Fig. 10.4

marathon runners, do die of heart attacks. One unfortunate example is James Fixx, a keen runner and the author of "The Complete Book of Running", who died of a heart attack aged 55. Unaccustomed exercise places the untrained cardiovascular system under sudden stress, and may actually cause heart attacks. Sedentary ex-sportsmen are especially vulnerable, launching themselves into training programmes similar to those they undertook 10–20 years earlier when they were fit. In snowy regions of North America and Europe, normally sedentary people often suffer heart attacks while pushing or shovelling out their snowbound cars.

Perhaps the best summary which can be given of this subject is to quote parts of two editorials:

'The proposal that marathon running could confer "immunity" to atherosclerosis now firmly belongs to the realm of cardiomythology.' *Lancet*, 3 December 1983.
and,
'Indeed, the evidence in favour of exercise is now so strong that we should no longer be defining the indications but the contraindications.' *British Medical Journal*, 7 January 1984.

While there is some evidence that endurance training may be beneficial to the cardiovascular system and may lessen the risk of coronary heart disease, the case is far from proven. Any fitness training programme should be approached with caution and moderation, particularly by the middle-aged. It may end up causing the very heart attack it was intended to prevent.

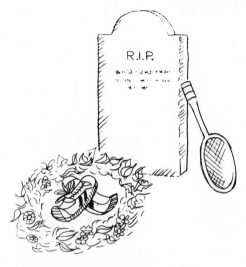

Fig. 10.5

High blood pressure (hypertension) and exercise

In the industrialised societies of Europe, America, and Australasia, the mean blood pressure of the population, expressed in milli-meters of mercury, is 120/80 (see Ch. 6, p. 111). If the blood pressures of a large number of people are measured carefully, a spectrum of values is obtained, some higher and others lower than the average, but there is no specific pressure which can clearly be labelled hypertensive. One rule-of-thumb suggests that systolic blood pressure should be 100 plus the person's age in years. Most doctors agree that people with blood pressures of over 160/95 should be treated. However, some doctors treat patients with pressures as low as 140/90, but there is little evidence that drug treatment of this group is beneficial.

blood pressure in exercise

During exercise, the demand for blood in working muscle increases. Cardiac output rises to meet this demand, by increasing the heart rate and the amount of blood pumped per stroke (see p. 128). Discharging a larger volume of blood into the arteries at each stroke increases systolic pressure (the pressure during the heart's pumping stroke). Since working muscles create a demand for blood flow by dilating their arteries, their resistance to flow is greatly reduced. Where large muscle groups are working (as in running), the flow resistance can drop to 20% of the resting value. Under these circumstances blood flows rapidly out of the arteries between beats reducing the diastolic pressure. Thus, in running the blood presssure might be 200/60 — a high systolic coupled with low diastolic pressure.

In the moderately hypertensive, exercise also raises the systolic blood pressure. However, several experiments have shown that the systolic pressure in exercise is similar to that seen in normotensive subjects. This suggests that exercise does not unduly strain the hearts of people with moderate hypertension. On the contrary, the low diastolic pressure characteristic of exercise actually reduces the load on the heart.

post-exercise blood pressure

After exercise the demand for blood flow gradually drops, as does the output of the heart. The systolic pressure falls rapidly, often to below normal resting values. The diastolic pressure also stays low. Sub-normal blood pressures are maintained for several hours after exercise. In moderate hypertension the magnitude of the post-exercise decrease in pressure can be large, often giving several hours of normal blood pressure without medication.

This effect is sufficiently reliable to be of real value. In countries where many people take out life or health insurance, individuals

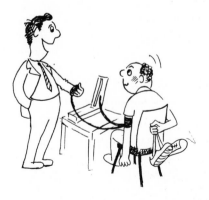

Fig. 10.6 An hour's running or similar activity reduces blood pressure for several hours.

with high blood pressures are penalised with high premiums. An hour's run before the medical examination may lower blood pressure by enough to avoid a surcharge!

It has been suggested that, due to this effect, regular vigorous exercise may usefully reduce blood pressure and might avoid the need for a lifetime of medication. The evidence for this is mixed, and people who remain physically active into middle age do not seem to have lower blood pressures than comparable sedentary individuals. However, active people also tend to be leaner, smoke less, and eat "healthier" diets than sedentary comparison groups, making it hard to realistically compare the two.

In summary, the various effects of regular physical activity ought to protect against coronary heart disease. Thus, exercise tends to alter the amount and composition of blood lipids in a protective direction. Although exercise alone does not cause obese people to lose weight (see p. 238), regular exercise tends to replace fatty tissue with muscle, slightly reducing obesity. Prolonged exercise decreases blood pressure and this effect is greatest in people with higher pressures. Frequent episodes of prolonged activity ought therefore to reduce blood pressure throughout the day. However, there is no evidence that fit, active individuals who train regularly have lower blood pressures than similar groups of sedentary people. Finally, there is no convincing evidence that groups of people who exercise regularly have fewer heart attacks than sedentary people, particularly if one corrects for differences in body weight, diet, smoking, etc.

Overtraining and the heart — Refer to Ch. 6, p. 141.

Osteoporosis and exercise

The literal translation of osteoporosis is porous bones. The bones of individuals with this condition are eroded, weakened and more likely to develop fractures than those of normal people. These fractures occur mainly in the lower spine and in the hip. Osteoporosis is largely a disease of post-menopausal women and it has been estimated that 25% of the American female population over the age of 60 suffer from it to some degree.

After the menopause, most women enter negative calcium balance. This means that they lose more calcium from their body than they absorb in their diet. For the majority of women the rate of loss is slow. The skeleton, the body's main store of calcium, is so large that death occurs before most women experience any symptoms. Osteoporosis may occur as a consequence of Cushing's disease (too much of the hormone cortisone), treatment with anti-inflammatory steroid drugs, and in certain forms of renal disease.

the standard treatment

Since osteoporosis is caused by the loss of calcium from the skeleton, logic suggests that it might be cured by simply giving extra dietary calcium. Unfortunately, dietary calcium therapy has little effect on the calcium balance of post-menopausal women. Moreover, a survey comparing the average calcium intake of women in various countries with the occurrence of fractures found no relationship. The United States and New Zealand, where the diet supplies one gram of calcium each day, had the highest indicence of fractures, while Hong Kong women had one third the number of fractures and less than half of the calcium intake.

Testosterone, the male sex hormone, promotes the rebuilding of bone and seems to protect men from osteoporosis. Treatment with testosterone is effective, but produces a number of side effects which are undesirable in women. Oestrogen, a female sex hormone, is also used as a treatment for osteoporosis. However, oestrogen doesn't always arrest calcium loss, and never promotes the rebuilding of bone. On the other hand, oestrogen is already widely used to treat post-menopausal women for other symptoms, and partial reversal of osteoporosis is a useful side-effect. Despite its limited effectiveness, oestrogen is a common prescription for osteoporosis. Recently small doses of another hormone, calcitonin, have been given together with oestrogen, and the combination seems to be more successful than oestrogen on its own.

It has been suggested that the best prevention of post-menopausal osteoporosis is to ensure that all women obtain adequate supplies of calcium in their youth. This will build strong, well mineralised bones which can tolerate calcium loss later in life, particularly if this loss can be slowed by hormone therapy. This attractive theory is unproven. In North America where the intake of milk has been high for decades, osteoporosis is a problem. On the other hand, traditional Oriental diets have long excluded dairy foods giving low calcium intakes, but osteoporosis is uncommon in these countries.

effects of physical activity

Bone demineralisation and weakening is not confined to post-menopausal women. Over 25 years ago, several groups of researchers showed that the density of bone in 50-year-old subjects depends on their habitual physical activity. Patients who are bedridden or immobile for any reason lose bone calcium. Calcium loss is also a problem for astronauts. Deprived of the constant stress imposed by gravity, their bones rapidly lose density and weaken. However, the skeleton is restored when normal stresses are reimposed. In other words, activity seemed to be the key to maintaining skeletal strength. For bedridden patients the answer is a speedy return to mobility. For astronauts, cramped accommodation and the absence of gravity, against which so much of the body's work is done, makes this difficult. Special exercise regimes using elastic and frictional loads have been devised for astronauts, but these are only partially effective.

effects of exercise in post-menopausal women

If activity stimulates growth and development of the skeleton, perhaps a deliberate increase in activity could reverse calcium loss. This simple hypothesis was recently tested by several Canadian

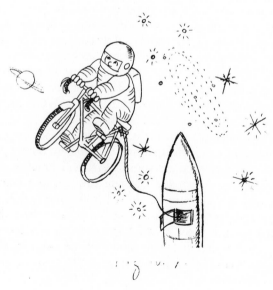

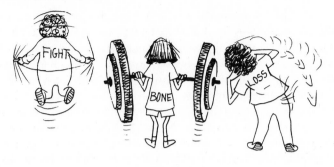

Fig. 10.8

doctors who studied the effects of supervised exercise (30 min/day, three times per week) on the bone density of a group of sedentary post-menopausal women. After one year bone density increased in the exercising women, while the control group who did little or no exercise showed no change.

The women attended aerobic dance sessions designed to raise their heart rate to 80% of their age-adjusted maximum. Although high, this is not an unrealistic level of exercise for sedentary women. In addition to increasing bone density, the aerobic capacity of these women improved by a dramatic 25%. This newly developed physical fitness is also likely to reduce fatigue, improve co-ordination, and produce a sensation of well-being. These alone are worthwhile results, which should encourage continued physical activity.

effects of vigorous exercise
Many people believe that if something is good, then more is probably better. One might expect to find particularly well mineralised bones in the very active. A recent study compared bone density in matched groups of young athletes and sedentary women, and surprisingly found no difference. A possible explanation is that there may be no such thing as a truly sedentary teenager, and the non-athletes were probably active enough to adequately stimulate bone mineralisation.

On the other hand, another study looked at two groups of young athletes, one group which was not menstruating and the other which was normal. Both groups were similar in age, weight, diet, and other characteristics, except that the amenorrheic (not menstruating) athletes ran twice as far in their weekly training as did the comparison group. The amenorrheic women had spinal vertebrae with 15% lower density than those of the menstruating group. The amenorrheic women also had far lower blood concentrations of oestrogen and progesterone.

Champion female endurance athletes are often amenorrheic. Evidently, the degree of training required to be a successful endurance athlete often causes amenorrhea, and a low rate of oestrogen and progesterone production — similar to that seen in postmenopausal women. Vigorous activity in these young athletes has clearly failed to protect them from bone loss. Protection may require a minimum oestrogen production, which was not achieved by these women.

The mechanism underlying this effect is not known, but it appears to be governed by the relative amounts of fat and muscle in the body. Extreme leanness in a woman, regardless of cause, always results in infertility associated with a lack of oestrogen and progesterone. Champion endurance athletes are very lean, and the females are often amenorrheic. Female body builders also strive for leanness in order to achieve good muscle definition, and are often amenorrheic. In both groups, a slackening of the training regime rapidly restores the production of sex hormones, normal menstruation and fertility.

possible effects of chronic amenorrhea

Many female athletes remain amenorrheic for years as a direct result of their sport or activity. This includes long distance runners, dancers, body builders, and others who gain an advantage from leanness or low body weight. Understandably, these people feel that their performance might be jeopardised by even the small weight gain which would allow them to resume menstruating. (Some women also feel that they perform less well when menstruating, although there is no evidence to support this.)

Young female athletes with amenorrhea may incorporate less calcium than normal into their skeletons. Their diminished calcium store may put them at increased risk of osteoporosis in later years when they begin to lose calcium during the menopause. This hypothesis, however, remains unproven.

the case of the female dancer

Today, dancers are athletes. Modern dancing technique often requires female dancers to become airborne, and also asks their male partners to lift them. Light weight has become a desirable feature particularly since it helps the male dancer to look strong and graceful. The dictates of modern fashion tend to reinforce this practical consideration. Nobody forces a female dancer to stay slim, but she certainly knows that promotion from the corps de ballet is unlikely if she becomes buxom or heavy.

Accordingly, many female dancers, in an attempt to retain a slim, immature shape, eat little relative to the metabolic requirements of their strenuous occupation. Their ability to sustain high levels of physical activity on a very modest energy intake is truly remarkable. Absent or irregular menstrual periods probably don't worry them. Amenorrhea may even be a bonus to an active person who clearly has no desire to become pregnant!

In recent years, there has been almost an epidemic of stress fractures in the bones of female dancers. Investigation shows that the mineral density of their bones is lower than that of non-dancers. At a time when most teenage girls are growing and laying down calcium in their skeletons, young dancers are failing to do so, and may be storing up for themselves an adulthood of osteoporosis.

summary

For a number of years there has been good evidence that inactivity is associated with bone calcium loss and that this is reversed by exercise, or merely by the resumption of normal activity. This applies to bedridden patients, astronauts, and athletes forced by injury into inactivity. Surprisingly, excessive activity in female athletes appears to also cause bone calcium loss, and this is associated with amenorrhea and very low rates of oestrogen and progesterone secretion, particularly when coupled with a low energy intake.

In post-menopausal women, calcium loss is also associated with a lack of oestrogen, and oestrogen replacement therapy partially relieves the problem. However, exercise therapy appears to increase the calcium content of bone, and is potentially capable of restoring normal bone density in older women. It is important to keep in mind that the amount of exercise required to produce this effect is realistic, and that the patient may also experience other benefits.

Obesity and exercise

An American scientist recently estimated that one third of the population of the United States is "too fat". On average, obese Americans are about 12 kilogrammes (25 pounds) overweight. The scientist went on to say that if it were possible to convert the fat carried by these people into motor fuel, this could power one million vehicles for a year! Americans are not unique. Obesity is a health problem in most developed countries. Blame can be assigned both to the proliferation of fast food shops tempting people to eat at all hours, and to the mechanisation of many tasks which once required human muscle.

Although not usually thought of as a disease, obesity is recognised as a health hazard. Aside from such obvious problems as overloaded joints, obesity increases the risk of hypertension, coronary heart disease, diabetes mellitus, renal disease, respiratory problems and gallstones. In addition, should surgery become necessary the thickness of fat can make the surgeon's job difficult. Anaesthetising obese patients is also dangerous because many anaesthetics dissolve in fat, and the dose is far harder to judge than in lean people. With a few exceptions (such as Sumo wrestlers) obesity is not admired in most societies, placing a psychological burden on fat people. Less importantly, obesity hampers movement, heat loss, and must reduce the enjoyment of life.

In the simplest terms, obesity is the result of an imbalance between energy intake (food) and energy expenditure (metabolic rate) (Ch. 3). Any difference between the two will cause body weight to change. If intake exceeds expenditure, energy will be stored as fat. There are no miracle cures. To lose weight, energy expenditure must exceed intake, however this condition may be achieved.

exercise and metabolic rate
Since exercise increases the metabolic rate, it seems almost obvious that it should also result in weight loss. However, putting this simple theory into practice has disappointed many people.

Energy expenditure during activity depends on the intensity of activity and also on body weight. The heavier the body, the more energy is required to move it. In one minute of vigorous exercise the human body burns 0.2 kilocalories (kcal) for each kilogram of body weight. Since the daily food intake is about 2400 kcal for men and 1800 for women, a great many minutes of work are needed to make a serious impression. The marathon is probably the maximum realistic amount of exercise one can do in a day. This burns an average day's energy intake in about three hours. However, most marathon runners will do nothing else that day and little on the following day or two apart from soaking sore feet. Marathons are not a sensible option for the average mortal.

In one hour of energetic basketball, football or hockey, a person might use a quarter of a day's energy intake. However, few people participate in an hour's sport every day. Years ago, many occupations (baker, lumberjack, agricultural labourer, sawyer, blacksmith, navvy, etc.) required a high rate of energy expenditure every day. Today, the widespread mechanisation of labour and transport offers little opportunity to burn energy at work, and even very active individuals generally burn far more energy while sedentary than they use during training or sports (see Table 3.2, p. 37).

can exercise cause weight to be lost?

Surely, any amount of exercise must increase energy expenditure and tilt the energy balance towards weight loss. If a person sets out to lose weight, they expect to lose fat, not muscle. In fact, this is not possible and lost weight is always a combination of fat and lean (protein, partly muscle) tissue.

When metabolised: 1 gram of fat yields 9 kcal,
and 1 gram of protein yields 4 kcal.

However, human tissues contain a lot of water:

fat tissue is 15% water (85% fat)
lean tissue is 80% water (20% protein)

and the energy value of fat tissue is $9 \times .85 = 7.7$ kcal/gram
the energy value of lean tissue is $4 \times .2 = 0.8$ kcal/gram.

Lean tissue loss can vary between 15% and 70% of the total weight loss, depending on the individual, their activity, and the diet followed. Assuming that the lost weight is 75% fat and 25% lean tissue (an unusually good result!), its energy value would be:

$(0.75 \times 7.7) + (0.25 \times 0.8) = 6.0$ calories per gram of weight lost.

As an example, consider a person weighing 100 kg (220 lbs or 15.7 st) wishing to lose 20 kg by vigorous exercise alone

at 6 kcal/gram, 20 kg is worth 12,000 kcal.

and vigorous exercise costs 0.2 kcal/kg/min, or 20 kcal/min for our subject.

Therefore, to lose the 20 kg would require a total of 600 minutes or 10 hours of vigorous exercise. Could our heavyweight shed the excess in ten weekly sessions of energetic sport, each lasting one hour?

why not?

Unfortunately, this approach is unlikely to work. There are several reasons why exercise alone is an impractical prescription for slimming:

1. Most overweight people are simply incapable of one hour's vigorous exercise. At best, they might accomplish 10–15 minutes of work at high intensity, or they could continue longer at a lighter load — perhaps four times as long. This should anyway be more effective (see below).

2. Clearly, if one wishes to lose fat, it is desirable to burn it as a fuel during exercise. On beginning exercise, the body initially obtains its energy almost exclusively from carbohydrate (see p. 54). Fat reserves are mobilised or removed from fat stores and carried in blood to the working muscles only gradually. It takes some thirty minutes of activity before fat begins to supply even half of the energy demand. Even at a modest work load, thirty minutes is beyond the endurance of many overweight people. To add insult to injury, the physically fit begin to use fat earlier than the overweight, and are able to supply a greater proportion of their energy demand from fat (see p. 58).

3. As work intensity increases, carbohydrate becomes the preferred source of energy. One advantage of being physically fit is the ability to use fat during high intensity activity. The fat are seldom fit, and unless the work load is relatively light, they derive most of their energy from carbohydrate. This makes it far harder for them to shed fat. Moreover, depletion of their glycogen stores demands replenishment. This cannot be done

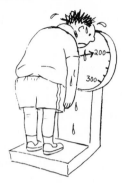

Fig. 10.9 Weight loss is seldom achieved by exercise alone.

from fat stores, only from the body's protein reserves or from food intake. This is one reason why exercise stimulates appetite — unfortunately more so in the overweight than in the physically fit!

4. Exercise builds muscles. If an overweight person embarks on a training programme, in due course they will become a fit overweight person, and well muscled beneath the fat. In effect, muscle begins to replace fat. However, if the intention was to become slim, this will not have been achieved.

In fact many experimental studies have shown that exercise on its own, without a reduction in food intake, results in no change, or only a small and disappointing drop in body weight. While exercise does raise energy expenditure, this increase is usually small compared to the normal day's metabolic requirement. Unless the diet is strictly controlled, food intake tends to increase and make up for the modest extra energy expenditure of exercise.

does this mean exercise is useless for weight loss?

In most people, body weight remains remarkably constant over many years. This is partly due to the efficient control of appetite so that hunger is suppressed unless the body requires food energy. Unfortunately, this control system is often overpowered by the temptations of modern life.

There is another system which helps us to maintain a constant body weight. The metabolic rate itself varies with food intake. In starvation, the metabolic rate falls by up to 30%. This response, of course, compounds the misery of the overweight. Tempted on all sides by advertisements for **FOOD**, and faced with an uncooperative bathroom scale which shows just how well their body has adapted to starvation, it is not surprising that so many fall by the wayside. To add further insult to injury, obese people seem to have a particularly efficient metabolism, with a lower than normal rate of energy expenditure.

Exercise can help. There is evidence that the decrease in metabolic rate on dieting is partly prevented by regular exercise.

Exercise also helps in another way. Simply reducing food intake reduces muscle mass as well as fat. In one experiment, with diet alone 40% of the weight lost was lean tissue. Adding a three mile daily walk had no effect on the total weight loss, but now only 25% of this was lean tissue, preserving muscle. The idea that the loss of lean tissue during dieting can be minimised by exercise has been confirmed in several studies.

In summary, exercise alone generally does not result in weight loss. However, coupled to a reduction in food intake, exercise often speeds weight loss, and ensures that more of the lost weight is fat rather than muscle.

Muscle damage caused by exercise

Physical activity can cause damage. Even in well trained athletes, high intensity training or competition can cause a variety of problems. For example, during running the feet strike the ground 1000 times per mile, with a force three times the body weight. This provides a lot of scope for injury, particularly when fatigue begins to affect co-ordination. Approximately 35% of all running injuries involve the knee, with less frequent problems in the foot and the hip. Although the pain associated with this damage should be a warning to stop, highly competitive amateurs and professional athletes often cannot afford to do so. Injections of anti-inflammatory steroids are sometimes given into joints, allowing injured athletes to continue in an important match or competition. Some athletes become so addicted to the euphoria associated with exercise that they may be virtually unaware of any pain.

Leaving aside relatively simple and obvious problems such

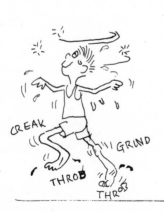

Fig. 10.10 Runners' "high" or euphoria may banish pain (see also Ch. 9, p. 219).

as tennis elbow, sprained ankle, and broken limbs, let us consider just muscle pain and damage.

muscle pain and damage

It is common knowledge that strenuous and prolonged activity can cause muscle pain severe enough to be crippling for days. Under the microscope, damaged muscle fibres are seen. This damage includes torn cell membranes, partial loss of the cell contents (enzymes, contractile proteins), various degrees of disorganisation of the contractile machinery, and invasion of the muscle cells by white blood cells associated with wounds and infections.

After strenuous activity, various substances normally found inside muscle cells can be detected in the blood. Since these substances are large protein molecules which normally do not cross the cell membrane, their presence in the blood is evidence that cell membranes have been damaged. In patients who are suspected of having suffered very mild heart attacks, the detection of these proteins in the blood (from damaged heart muscle) has long been taken as clinical proof that such an event has actually occurred.

As final evidence of muscle damage, there is loss of strength. Under appropriate conditions, the tension measured immediately after a damaging test exercise can be reduced to half or less of the pre-exercise value.

The degree of damage is directly proportional to the intensity of activity and its duration, and inversely proportional to the physical fitness of the individual. Thus, an athlete can engage in more vigorous activity than may a sedentary person before sustaining injury.

concentric v. eccentric contraction

Certain types of activity are far more likely to result in injury than others. In general, there are two kinds of muscle contraction. The first is concentric, where the contracting muscle shortens, and the second is eccentric, where the contracting muscle lengthens. Concentric muscle activity is the more common, and characteristic of most of our movement. Eccentric activity is experienced during running down stairs or lowering a weight on a rope, where muscle activity acts as a brake on movement generated by outside forces.

Muscles work less hard during eccentric activity and the subjective perception of effort is less than for concentric movement. The

243

amount of electrical activity in the nerves controlling the muscles is also lower for eccentric activity. Finally, muscles develop less tension during eccentric than in concentric activity. Nevertheless, eccentric contraction is far more likely to result in muscle damage and pain.

pain v. damage v. performance

It is logical to expect that pain, damage, and diminished performance following strenuous exercise should all occur together. However, while muscle performance is poorest shortly after the test exercise and steadily improves, the pain or soreness peaks at one to three days. On the other hand, the visible signs of muscle damage under the microscope are barely detectable on the first day, but peak after five to seven days. The blood concentrations of cellular proteins also peak at one week, supporting the microscopic evidence. The repair of even severely damaged muscle fibres is generally complete by three weeks.

The time separation between visible muscle damage and diminished ability to develop tension is confusing. Under the microscope damaged muscle fibres may have lost much of their contractile machinery one week after severe exercise, and there can be no doubt that these fibres could produce little tension. On the other hand, by this time muscle performance is already partly restored.

It is possible that subjects whose muscles are very sore cannot be relied upon to produce a test contraction of maximum effort. To avoid this problem and ensure accuracy, in some experiments muscle tension has been measured using external electrical stimu-

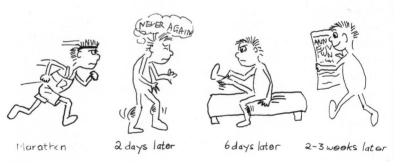

Fig. 10.11 *How soon one forgets.*

lation of the muscles so that the subject's discomfort cannot affect performance.

It is well known that, when a recently exercised subject is asked to contract a sore and damaged muscle, there is pain initially, which diminishes on continued activity. Several experimenters have also found that pain diminishes after five minutes of repetitive contraction and almost vanishes by fifteen minutes. Interestingly, in these tests, contraction strength was unchanged throughout, apparently unaffected by changes in the intensity of pain reported by the subjects.

Clearly, the relationships between muscle damage, pain, and the performance of previously overworked muscles are still poorly understood, as are the causes of these symptoms.

effects of training

In well trained individuals, the intensity of activity which may be undertaken without causing damage or pain is far greater than for sedentary people. If an eccentric exercise regime is undertaken by sedentary individuals several times at intervals of two weeks, pain, damage and performance loss is experienced each time. However, on the second and third repetitions, its extent is markedly reduced, showing that the test itself has a training effect.

There is no doubt that even training of mild intensity before the test exercise will markedly reduce the severity of symptoms. Thus, a person who bicycles to work — perhaps only three miles each day — suffers markedly fewer symptoms following a 100 mile day trip than another who cycles rarely.

recovery

Happily, recovery from the damage, pain, and diminished muscle performance is complete. The pain resolves rapidly, and is mostly gone within five days, although in some subjects it can take longer. Damage and pain are less and recovery is faster in trained than in sedentary subjects. The improved outlook for trained subjects may be partly due to the likelihood that they will be active during the recovery period.

There are a number of preparations on the market which are used by athletes to alleviate post-exercise trauma. These range from simple alcohol rubs to both steroidal and non-steroidal anti-inflammatory drugs. At this time, there is no evidence that any of these is genuinely effective in promoting or speeding healing. Despite this, many users are convinced that they do reduce pain and sales remain buoyant.

summary

Hard exercise causes pain, visible muscle damage (under the microscope), chemical evidence of this damage, and diminished muscle performance. Eccentric exercise, where the muscles work as brakes on movement imposed from outside, causes more pain than concentric work, where muscles initiate movement.

Reduced muscle performance is seen immediately on completion of the test exercise, and recovers steadily over the next ten days. Pain is rarely sensed until the following day, usually peaks on the second day, and vanishes within one week. Although there is some evidence of changes in muscle structure under the microscope on the day following exercise, visible damage peaks between the fifth and seventh day, when the various proteins spilled from the damaged muscle fibres reach their maximum concentration in the blood.

Recovery from muscle damage appears to be complete. The effects of exercise are less severe in trained than untrained individuals, and the amount of training required to acquire a useful degree of protection is surprisingly small. Trained individuals also recover more rapidly.

The message must be that the prospect of muscle pain and damage should not deter anyone from physical activity. Rather, everyone should maintain a reasonable level of physical fitness which will partly or completely shield them from the consequences of unexpected strenuous activity.

Heat exhaustion or heat stroke

The symptoms of heat exhaustion are very high body temperature during or following strenuous exertion. Surprisingly, in people undertaking endurance activity, this can occur at temperatures as low as 10°C. Heat exhaustion can also be brought on without exertion by severe dehydration. If nothing is done, it leads to collapse. Fainting may occur in the absence of either exertion or dehydration in people required to remain standing for some time.

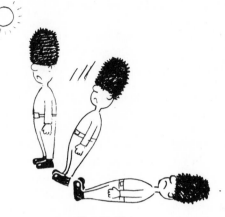

Fig. 10.12

This is related to heat exhaustion because it occurs most often in warm weather. A classic example is the red-coated Guardsman, at rigid attention in his bearskin hat and scarlet jacket, fainting outside Buckingham Palace.

Untreated, heat exhaustion can be fatal. The rise in body temperature is due to the inability of the cardiovascular system to deliver a sufficient blood flow to the skin to cool the body. If unchecked, body temperature may continue to rise and this could eventually cause irreversible brain damage.

what causes heat exhaustion?

During strenuous exercise large amounts of heat are produced, and this must be dissipated by the evaporation of sweat. To produce sweat, fluid is removed from the blood by the sweat glands to form a watery secretion. As sweat is lost, the volume of the blood plasma diminishes. In general, for each litre of sweat produced, the blood volume is reduced by half a litre (the remainder is taken from other body compartments).

The effect is somewhat like that of a haemorrhage. In response to the volume reduction, the pressure within the venous system decreases. This pressure returns blood to the heart, and as it drops the rate at which the heart can fill between beats diminishes. With less blood pumped at each beat, the heart rate tends to rise in an attempt to maintain the heart's output. One sign of the development of heat exhaustion is a steady increase in heart rate.

During sweating, water and some salts are lost, leaving behind blood with an increased concentration of red cells and plasma proteins. This water-depleted blood is also viscous or "thick", and circulates with more difficulty than does normal blood. For this reason, the loss of one litre of plasma volume as a result of sweating has a greater effect on cardiovascular performance than would the haemorrhage of a similar volume of whole blood.

As venous pressure decreases and blood viscosity increases, the output of the heart diminishes. It gradually becomes difficult to supply all of the blood flow demanded by the working muscles and the cardiovascular system begins to economise on the amount of blood sent to the skin. This is the primary reason for the overheating characteristic of heat exhaustion. Under normal conditions the victim becomes distressed, and slows down or stops.

dangers of heat exhaustion
A determined athlete may ignore the warnings. Continuing to work at a rate greater than a decreasing blood supply can support forces the cardiovascular system to divert blood flow from "unimportant" areas like the kidney, digestive system and skin to the working muscles. Since these muscles still receive less blood than they require, they move away from aerobic towards anaerobic metabolism to supply their energy. The production and accumulation of lactic acid in these now poorly supplied muscles eventually forces their blood vessels to dilate, lowering blood pressure and finally reducing blood flow to the brain. This is the immediate cause of collapse.

In "normal" fainting venous blood pools in the legs, failing to return to the heart, and blood pressure falls. In this case, collapse to the horizontal position returns the pooled venous blood to the heart restoring blood pressure, and the subject regains consciousness quickly. However, in collapse due to heat exhaustion there is no blood pooled in the legs, and the poor output of the heart is simply due to low blood volume. The horizontal position cannot return more blood to the heart although flow to the brain may improve somewhat. Low blood pressure is caused by blood vessels which are dilated because of excess waste product accumulation. These blood vessels have effectively escaped from the control of

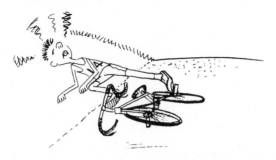

Fig. 10.13 Heat exhaustion during a sporting event can be dangerous.

the cardiovascular system. This failure to maintain a minimum blood pressure is termed "shock" (see p. 124).

Since collapse as a consequence of heat exhaustion barely improves cardiovascular performance, blood pressure remains low as does the blood flow to the skin. With its low rate of blood flow, the skin is unable to produce sweat. (One characteristic of heat exhaustion is a dry skin.) Since there is too little blood flow available to carry heat to the skin and too little sweat to cool it, heat dissipation almost stops.

"Explosive temperature rise" is the expression used to describe this consequence of heat exhaustion, and when this occurs, the victim is said to be suffering from "Heat Stroke". Since heat loss slows down while exertion may continue, the body temperature rises rapidly. Brain temperatures in excess of 41°C result in disorientation and contribute to the collapse of heat exhaustion. Confusion occurs in the short term but, if the individual is not cooled quickly, there may be permanent damage. Heat stroke is considered a medical emergency and is treated with heroic measures, sometimes even packing the patient in ice.

treatment
Treatment of heat exhaustion simply consists of cooling the victim to restore normal body temperature. If he/she is sufficiently conscious to swallow, water is administered to boost blood volume and dilute it towards normal values. If the temperature is brought under control rapidly, there will be a complete and rapid recovery.

heat cramp

Heat cramp is another problem associated with the production of large amounts of sweat. Heat cramp, heat exhaustion and fainting are all related to one another. The symptoms of heat cramp are uncontrolled and painful muscle contraction. These tend to occur after prolonged exertion in a warm environment when periodic drinking is possible. Heat cramp is not really harmful, although it can be very painful and is temporarily disabling.

During exercise, particularly in the heat, large quantities of sweat are produced. This sweat contains salt or sodium chloride which is thereby lost from the body. As water is consumed to replace the lost sweat, the body fluids are diluted, particularly with respect to sodium. It is thought that a reduced concentration of sodium is the underlying cause of heat cramp.

Salt tablets or some other form of salt supplement is the logical and preferred treatment for heat cramp. However, this may not be necessary, and complete recovery usually follows water replacement and rest. This suggests that the simple explanation given above may not be correct. Moreover, salt supplementation retards heat acclimatisation (see p. 188), and may increase the likelihood of future attacks of heat cramp.

Conclusion

At the beginning, a distinction was made between endurance and strength training. At the extreme, the results of these two types of training look very different. The endurance trained individual is generally lean, and may be lean to the point of appearing emaciated. The prototype of the strength trained person is heavily muscled, but also often lean.

There is no doubt that many of the consequences of regular exercise are beneficial. However, as with other things, exercise can be carried to extremes. Many of the consequences of overenthusiastic training are unpleasant, and some are dangerous. One is reminded of the sad story of the 17-year-old American, Mary Lou Retton, gymnastic gold medallist in the 1984 Olympics. By age 20 she was partly crippled with arthritis, apparently a consequence of intensive training before her joints were fully formed and capable of bearing heavy loads. The media are not inquisitive in Eastern Europe, and we do not know the fate of their young champion gymnasts. The case of Tracey Austin is similar. A contender for the women's tennis crown at Wimbledon when only 14, she suffered many injuries and faded from top competition before turning 20. Again, her injuries were attributed to excessive training before her skeleton was ready.

If not carried to excess, exercise is beneficial in a number of ways. Probably most useful is the feeling of energy and well being which a fit person enjoys. However, between commuting to a generally sedentary job and enjoying a few of the passive entertainments available, today's modern world offers little opportunity for exercise. The best solution must be to integrate activity into the daily routine, rather than to undertake energetic sports or training. With advancing age, enthusiasm for athletics wanes. However, once in the habit of bicycling or walking to work, or of using stairs instead of a lift, this activity is likely to continue throughout life. A useful level of physical fitness can be maintained, protecting the individual from the worst consequences of occasional heavy exertion, and endowing him or her with a satisfying degree of endurance and fatigue resistance — both essential to extract the maximum enjoyment out of life.

Appendix

Energy expenditure and heat production in various activities

| Activity | Males (75 kg) | | Females (60 kg) | |
	Energy cost (kcal/hr)	Heat output (watts)	Energy cost (kcal/hr)	Heat output (watts)
Rest	95	110	75	85
Clean, sweep	260	310	225	260
Brisk walk	360	420	290	335
Run (7 mph)	875	1,020	700	810
(10 mph)	1,130	1,310	950	1,100
Cycle (10 mph)	450	525	360	420
(16 mph)	765	890	615	715
Badminton	440	515	350	405
Tennis	495	575	400	460
Squash	755	875	760	890
Golf	385	445	310	360
Swimming (slow)	545	635	445	515
(fast)	695	810	565	660

The energy expenditures and rates of heat production in this table are only approximate because of body size, skill, and intensity of activity. The data in this table are intended to provide a rough idea of the caloric cost of various activities.

Additional reading

The books below are suggested reading for people who would like additional information. The first four are textbooks which cover the subject at greater length than was possible here. Their main disadvantage to the student of exercise physiology is cost. I found the first two to be particularly well written. For people who once knew physiology but have forgotten it or for students who would like a review, the fifth book is an excellent summary.

For those who believe that exercise is the cure for all of the world's ills, I recommend the sixth book which takes a very sceptical stand. Unfortunately for the author, his well presented arguments have been largely ignored in the current pro-exercise fervour. For those who believe that nutrition is the key to better performance, the seventh book is an elegantly written and very readable introduction to nutrition while the eighth provides authoritative information on nutrition for sportsmen. Finally, I recommend the last book for people who are tempted to "soup up" their performance by using drugs.

1. *Textbook of Work Physiology* by Per-Olof Astrand and Kaare Rodahl, McGraw Hill (1986, 3rd edn).
2. *Exercise Physiology* by William McArdle, Frank Katch and Victor Katch, Lea and Febiger (1986, 2nd edn).
3. *Physiology of Exercise* by David Lamb, Macmillan (1984, 2nd edn).
4. *Exercise Physiology* by George Brooks and Thomas Fahey, Wiley (1984).
5. *Color Atlas of Physiology* by A. Despopoulos and S. Silbernagl, Georg Thieme Verlag (1984, 2nd edn).
6. *The Exercise Myth* by Henry Solomon, Angus and Robertson (1985).
7. *Nutrition, Diet & Health* by Michael Gibney, Cambridge (1986).
8. *Nutrition for Sport* by Steve Wooton, Simon and Schuster (1986).
9. *Drugs in Sport* by D.R. Mottram, Spon (1988).

Glossary

A-V NODE
the atrio-ventricular node; bundle of tissue modified from heart muscle which conducts electrical excitation from the atria to the ventricles (across the layer of insulating tissue which separates them); A-V node delays the electrical signal allowing atrial systole to occur before ventricular systole begins

ACCLIMATISATION
the process of becoming accustomed to a new stress, for example: acclimatisation to a high altitude environment with stresses of cold, low oxygen pressure and dryness

ACETYLCHOLINE
substance released from certain nerves which slows the heart and generally dilates blood vessels; its release from nerve endings on skeletal muscle cells excites them, causing contraction

ACTIN
contractile protein found in muscle; the thin filaments are composed of actin

ACTION POTENTIAL
positive voltage "spike" accompanying cellular excitation in muscle and nerve cells

ADENOSINE TRIPHOSPHATE (ATP)
substance which readily loses one or two phospates (becoming first adenosine diphosphate — ADP, and then adenosine monophosphate — AMP), thereby releasing chemical energy to power most of the body's activities;

ADP
Adenosine diphosphate — see ADENOSINE TRIPHOSPHATE

ADRENALINE
adrenal gland hormone which stimulates the heart and causes most blood vessels to relax (see also NORADRENALINE)

AEROBIC (METABOLISM)
literally "with oxygen" — refers to the formation of ATP by all metabolic processes except glycolysis (anaerobic metabolism)

AEROBIC THRESHOLD
the work load or rate at which an appreciable amount of the energy required is provided by anaerobic processes; usually defined as the

work load at which the lactic acid concentration in the blood rises to 4 mmol/litre (see also OBLA)

AMATEUR

literally a sportsman who plays or competes for the love of a sport; today, true amateurs are hard to find amongst the top ranks of Olympic participants

AMINO ACIDS

small molecules composed of carbon, hydrogen and nitrogen which link together to form PROTEINS; the building blocks of living matter

AMP

Adenosine monophosphate — see ADENOSINE TRIPHOSPHATE

AMPHETAMINE

a stimulant which reduces sleepiness and suppresses appetite; used by sportsmen to reduce fatigue and improve endurance; amphetamine's effectiveness is widely believed but unproven

ANABOLIC (METABOLISM)

the biological manufacture of complex substances from simple molecules; generally referring to the synthesis of protein from amino acids (see TESTOSTERONE)

ANAEROBIC (METABOLISM)

"without oxygen" — refers to the formation of ATP by GLYCOLYSIS, which requires no oxygen

ANALGESICS

pain relieving drugs, eg. aspirin, codeine

ANGINA

intense and frightening pain associated with an inadequate oxygen supply to the heart muscle; probably caused by narrowed coronary arteries restricting blood (and oxygen) supply to the heart; sometimes occurs during exercise, sometimes during periods of anxiety, sometimes even at rest

AORTA

the large artery conducting blood away from the left side of the heart to supply the body

ARTERIOLE

small muscular high pressure blood vessel

ARTERY

elastic high pressure blood vessel

ATP — see ADENOSINE TRIPHOSPHATE

ATRIO-VENTRICULAR VALVES

separate the atria from the ventricles — tricuspid valve on the right side, mitral valve on the left

ATRIUM

thin-walled, low pressure pumping chambers of the heart (two — left and right)

BARORECEPTORS
arterial devices the body uses for measuring blood pressure
BASAL METABOLIC RATE — see METABOLIC RATE
BETA-BLOCKERS
a class of drug used for the treatment of hypertension working by preventing some of the actions of adrenalin and noradrenalin; used in precision sports like shooting where by reducing tremor and stroke volume they improve accuracy
BLOOD PLASMA
the fluid in which the red blood cells are bathed containing dissolved electrolytes (mainly sodium, chloride, and bicarbonate with smaller amounts of calcium and potassium), and plasma proteins (mainly albumins and globulins)
BLOOD PRESSURE
usually arterial pressure — the pressure measured by the doctor — normally 120/80 mmHg (systolic/diastolic)
BLOOD VOLUME
the volume of the circulatory system, usually 45% red cells in man, 40% in woman
BODY FLUIDS
the fluids of which the body is composed — the INTRACELLULAR FLUID and the EXTRACELLULAR FLUID, the latter subdivided into the INTERSTITIAL FLUID and the BLOOD PLASMA
CAFFEINE
a stimulant present in coffee, tea and other beverages; said to improve endurance performance; effectiveness in sport widely believed but unproven
CALCIUM
a metallic element and an essential element; release of calcium ions into the cell triggers some cell activities; bone is made up of poorly soluble salts of calcium
CALORIE
a unit of heat and energy; the amount of heat required to raise the temperature of one gram of water by one centigrade degree; scientifically the unit has been replaced by the Joule — 4.186 Joules = 1 Calorie; kilocalories are used to measure the food energy intake
CAPILLARY
very fine blood vessel where exchange of materials between blood and tissues occurs
CARBOHYDRATES
a family of compounds of carbon, hydrogen and oxygen which are commonly found in starchy foodstuffs such as roots (potatoes, carrots) and grains (wheat, rice) and in sweet foods

CARBON DIOXIDE
the major gaseous product of metabolism (and of burning); a gas which, dissolved in water, forms carbonic acid (a weak acid); the metabolic product which most directly controls the vigour of breathing

CARDIAC CYCLE
time required for a complete contraction and relaxation cycle of the heart; the reciprocal of heart rate

CARDIAC MUSCLE
the type of muscle found in the heart; striated like skeletal muscle, but with some of the properties of smooth muscle (see also SMOOTH, and SKELETAL MUSCLE)

CARDIAC OUTPUT
the total amount of blood pumped by each side of the heart per minute; equal to the VENOUS RETURN

CATABOLIC (METABOLISM)
breakdown of complex substances into simpler molecules

CENTRAL CARDIOVASCULAR CONTROL
the control of blood flow is shared between the brain (central control) and local mechanisms (see LOCAL CONTROL)

CHOLESTEROL
fatty molecule bearing a close resemblance to the steroid hormones and present in all cell membranes; a major constituent of the atherosclerotic plaques which occur in arteries; excessive cholesterol in the blood is associated with coronary heart disease
HDL CHOLESTEROL — the portion of blood cholesterol present as High Density Lipoprotein, and thought to be "beneficial" as distinct from
LDL CHOLESTEROL — the portion of blood cholesterol present as Low Density Lipoprotein, and thought to be "harmful"

CHROMATOGRAPHY
a method of chemical analysis in which a sample to be analysed moves over or through a stationary material which absorbs and detains the passage of various substances, thereby separating the components of the sample

COCAINE
a stimulant traditionally taken in small doses by Andean natives; in large doses highly addictive; improves endurance by reducing the sensation of pain and discomfort

COLD-BLOODED
a misnomer for animals which can only warm themselves by absorbing heat from the environment; certain "cold-blooded" reptiles maintain daytime temperatures well over 30°C! (see also WARM-BLOODED)

COLLAGEN
> tough protein material within the blood vessels which strengthens them, limiting stretch; also present in cartilage and tendons

CONCENTRIC (CONTRACTION)
> a contraction during which muscle shortening occurs — by far the most common type of contraction (see ECCENTRIC)

CONDUCTION
> the transfer of heat between regions of different temperature by means of the exchange of kinetic energy between molecules; the rate of heat conduction depends on the thermal conductivity of the material, the total surface area through which heat is passing, and the temperature gradient

CONTRACTION
> the activation and shortening of muscle (for heart, see SYSTOLE)

CONVECTION
> the transfer of heat between regions of different temperature within a fluid by fluid movement (eg. hot fluid moves to cool region); depends on the rate of flow, the heat capacity of the fluid, the surface area of contact, and the temperature gradient

COUNTERCURRENT HEAT EXCHANGE
> a scheme whereby heat is lost from a warm fluid moving in one direction and gained by a cold fluid moving in the opposite direction; suitably organised, the cold fluid leaving the system can nearly attain the temperature of the warm fluid entering (and vice versa) (see Ch. 7, Fig. 7.12)

CREATINE PHOSPHATE (PCr)
> substance which readily loses its phosphate, thereby releasing energy to power the regeneration of ATP from ADP or AMP (see ADENOSINE TRIPHOSPHATE); forms a store of energy backing up the primary store of "instantaneous" energy, ATP; also called phosphocreative (PCr)

> water or fluid loss; a sufficiently large loss can reduce the volume of blood the heart can pump; the loss of 10% of the body's weight threatens survival

DEPOLARISE
> to remove polarity; cell membranes are polarised with their inside negative relative to the outside, when depolarised, this voltage difference is reduced, often exciting the cell

DIASTOLE
> period of cardiac cycle when the ventricles are filling or "resting"

DIASTOLIC PRESSURE
> the arterial blood pressure during diastole (between beats), when the ventricles are relaxed — normally 80 mmHg

DIURETICS
a group of drugs used to treat oedema and hypertension, which greatly
increase urine volume; used by boxers, jockeys, etc. to "make weight"
before competition

ECCENTRIC (CONTRACTION)
a contraction during which the muscle lengthens — occurs during
braking eg. walking downhill, or lowering a weight on a rope (see
CONCENTRIC)

ECG (EKG)
electrocardiogram — recording of the electrical activity of the heart

EFFICIENCY
a comparison between the useful output which can be obtained from a
process and the magnitude of input required to make it work

ELASTIN
protein material within blood vessels which gives them elasticity,
allowing them to resist stretch

ELECTROLYTE
substance which, dissolved in water, dissociates (splits) into positively
and negatively charged particles; usually salts like sodium chloride
(table salt)

ENDORPHINES
opium-like substances formed naturally in the brain under conditions
of stress; produce a mild euphoria and analgesia lasting several hours

ENDOTHELIAL CELL
smooth, slippery cells with anti-clotting properties lining the entire
cardiovascular system (and other tissues)

ENDURANCE
ability to continue a given activity

ENERGY EXPENDITURE
the rate at which energy is consumed by the body (or metabolic rate);
usually expressed as kilocalories per minute or per day

EPHEDRINE
a stimulant with actions similar to AMPHETAMINE

ERGOMETER
literally "work measurer"; a device to measure the rate at which work
is done; commonly bicycle ergometers and treadmills, although rowing
and swimming ergometers also exist, and even a dinghy ergometer has
been devised to estimate work output while sailing

EVAPORATION
the process of changing the state of a substance from liquid to gas
which requires energy; the evaporation of water requires about
550 Calories or 2300 Joules of heat for each gram of water
vapourised

K

EXTRACELLULAR FLUID
all of the fluid outside the body's cells and approximately equal to 21% of the body's weight in men and 16% in women

FAST TWITCH MUSCLE
large skeletal muscle fibres specialised for anaerobic, sprint activity

FATIGUE
the inability to maintain performance in activity

FATS
a family of compounds of carbon, hydrogen and small amounts of oxygen which are commonly found in meat, and which can be extracted from certain vegetable foods (maize, olives, palm nuts)

FIBRIL (MYOFIBRIL)
chains of sarcomeres; a muscle cell is composed of hundreds of myofibrils

FILAMENT (MYOFILAMENT)
contractile proteins in muscle are formed into very fine filaments of actin and myosin

FILTRATION
pressure within the cardiovascular system causes some fluid to ooze (filter) out of capillaries — filtration is limited by the osmotic pressure exerted by plasma proteins (see OEDEMA and OSMOTIC PRESSURE)

FULCRUM
pivot point of a lever

GLYCOGEN
the form in which carbohydrate is stored in animals — "animal starch"; two thirds of the body's glycogen is found in its muscles, and one third in the liver

GLYCOLYSIS
breakdown of glucose molecule (six carbon atoms) into two pyruvate molecules (three carbons), which simultaneously regenerates two ATPs from two ADPs (see ANAEROBIC)

GROWTH HORMONE (GH)
a protein hormone and very species specific (rat GH doesn't work in mice and pig GH doesn't work in man) which controls growth before puberty; can substitute for anabolic steroids in athletes if price and availability are no object

HAEMOGLOBIN
iron-containing molecule specialised for the transport of oxygen; red blood cells are filled with haemoglobin, which gives blood its red colour

HAEMORRHAGE
loss of blood volume

HEART BLOCK
    failure of excitation transmission from atrium to ventricle — ventricles
    and atria beat independently
HORMONES
    substances secreted by endocrine glands to regulate body processes by
    either stimulating or inhibiting the functions of groups of cells
HYPERTENSION
    high blood pressure; worth treating when the systolic pressure is higher
    than 160 mmHg and the diastolic pressure is higher than 95 mmHg
HYPERTHERMIA
    a body temperature well in excess of the normal value; a temperature
    of 40°C or higher would be called hyperthermia
HYPERTROPHY
    increase in a tissue (often muscle) due to increased size of cells
INSULIN
    a protein hormone which acts to reduce the blood glucose (sugar)
    concentration by encouraging tissues to remove glucose from blood
INTERSTITIAL WATER
    the fluid in which the cells are bathed; mostly the EXTRACELLULAR
    fluid minus the plasma volume
INTRACELLULAR FLUID
    the fluid contained within the body's cells and approximately equal to
    43% of the body's weight in men and and 34% in women
ION
    a charged particle in solution; on dissolving, electrolytes split up into
    two or more charged particles, with equal numbers of positive and
    negative charges; for example, when calcium chloride dissolves, one
    calcium ion with two positive charges and two chloride ions with one
    negative charge each are formed — the process is written as follows:
    $CaCl_2 \rightarrow Ca^{++} + 2Cl^-$ (see ELECTROLYTE)
ISOMETRIC
    in Greek, "equal length"; in isometric muscle contraction little
    movement takes place eg. straining against opposite sides of a
    doorway; in practice, muscle contractions in which tension is high and
    movement slight eg. weight lifting
ISOTONIC
    in Greek, "equal tension"; in isotonic muscle contraction, movement is
    great but little tension is developed eg. running on the level
JOULE
    a unit of work, heat and energy; defined as the work done when either
    (a) a force of 1 Newton acts over a distance of 1 Metre, or (b) an
    electric current of 1 Ampére flows through a resistance of 1 Ohm; one

Joule of work for one second is equivalent to one Watt of power (see
also CALORIE and WATT)

LACTIC ACID
product of ANAEROBIC metabolism which can accumulate during
hard work; also called lactate

LOCAL CONTROL
blood flow is partly controlled by the accumulation of metabolic waste
products within a tissue, which dilates its blood vessels (see CENTRAL
CARDIOVASCULAR CONTROL)

MEMBRANE (CELL)
a thin, structured film of mostly fatty material with some protein
present which separates the contents of the cell from the fluid
surrounding it; cell membranes are generally PERMEABLE to some
materials and impermeable to others

MEMBRANE POTENTIAL
small voltage across the membranes of all living cells (inside always
negative); 70–100 millivolts in muscle and nerve, lower in other tissues

METABOLIC RATE
rate (varying) at which the body uses energy; generally estimated from
the rate at which oxygen is used; The BASAL METABOLIC RATE is
the lowest rate of energy expenditure, measured eight hours after the
last meal and after 1–2 hours of complete rest

METABOLISM
a set of interlinked chemical reactions by which the living body extracts
energy from foodstuffs or stores and uses it for all of its activities: to
produce heat; for movement; to maintain a constant internal
environment; to build protein, bone, etc; for reproduction ...

MITOCHONDRION (plural — Mitochondria)
organelle found in most cells; where aerobic metabolism takes place

MOTOR UNIT
a motor nerve cell and the skeletal muscle cells it controls; motor
nerves always contol a number of muscle cells — up to 1000 muscle
fibres in postural muscles, as few as five muscle fibres in muscles of the
eye and hand

MYOFIBRIL (see FIBRIL)

MYOFILAMENT (see FILAMENT)

MYOGLOBIN
approximately one quarter of the haemoglobin molecule and found
mainly in red or slow twitch muscle (and responsible for its dark
colour); its presence increases the rate of oxygen diffusion in the muscle

MYOSIN
contractile protein found in muscle; the thick filaments are composed
of myosin

NERVE CELL (NEURON)
a cell equipped with a number of thread-like processes (up to 1 m long) making contact with other cells; highly specialised for information transmission by means of action potentials travelling at 20–120 m/sec.

NEUROTRANSMITTER
a chemical substance released by a nerve cell, which diffuses across the tiny gap separating two cells and excites the neighbouring cell

NORADRENALINE
an adrenal gland hormone (also produced by some nerves) which stimulates the heart and also causes most blood vessels to constrict (see ADRENALINE)

OBESITY
excessive fatness; various tables exist defining obesity by age and sex

OBLA (ONSET OF BLOOD LACTATE)
a human performance test which determines the work rate at which lactic acid begins to accumulate in the blood; OBLA is an index of the maximum continuous work rate, or "cruising speed" of an individual; endurance training can improve OBLA markedly (see VO_{2MAX}); (see also ANAEROBIC THRESHOLD)

OEDEMA
swelling due to the excessive accumulation of extracellular fluid; often due to capillary injury causing leakage of plasma protein which is accompanied by plasma fluid (see FILTRATION and OSMOTIC PRESSURE)

OSMOTIC PRESSURE
If two solutions are separated by a membrane which is permeable to the solvent but not to the solute, fluid will move from the less concentrated to the more concentrated solution. Osmotic pressure is the pressure which must be applied to prevent this movement (called osmosis). In blood, plasma proteins supply most of the osmotic pressure which prevents plasma from leaking out of the capillaries.

OSTEOPOROSIS
disease of "porous bones" which occurs when bone loses some of its mineral content; most frequent in post-menopausal women

OXYGEN DEBT
refers to the degree by which the oxygen consumption lags behind the true "oxygen cost" of an activity, and to the period of elevated oxygen consumption which continues after activity has stopped; although sounding as if "borrowed" oxygen is being paid back (and originally thought to be this), it is really due to a persistently elevated metabolic rate

PACEMAKER
a small bundle of modified heart muscle cells in the right atrium whose

spontaneous electrical activity excites the neighbouring heart muscle; this rhythmic discharge is responsible for the heart beat (see S-A NODE) ARTIFICIAL — if the pacemaker malfunctions (eg. heart block), an electronic device is implanted which maintains regular ventricular contraction

PCr (see CREATINE PHOSPHATE)

PERICARDIUM

a thin, tough, inelastic membrane closely enclosing the heart, and limiting its volume increase when the venous pressure rises; protects the heart from volume increase (temporarily) during heart failure

PERIPHERAL RESISTANCE

total resistance to flow offered by the blood vessels — an increase reduces blood flow; blood flow to all tissues is regulated by individual adjustments in flow resistance (by ARTERIOLES)

PERMEABLE

allowing penetration; a MEMBRANE allowing certain substances to pass through is said to be PERMEABLE to these, but impermeable to those materials it excludes; generally cell membranes are permeable to potassium ions but not to sodium ions

PHYSICAL FITNESS

the state of being able to carry out a physically demanding task; physical fitness can be tested by competition, but is generally judged in a more casual manner; it is impossible to attain universal fitness, but training for the modern decathlon probably comes as close as possible to this ideal; for the ordinary mortal, fitness might be defined as the ability to carry out whatever activities one enjoys or has to do, without painful consequences

POTASSIUM

the major positive ION found inside cells

POWER

power is the rate at which work is done; in physiology, "work rate" is often abbreviated to simply "work"; the work rate is commonly expressed in Watts, where one Watt = one Joule per second (see WORK)

PRE-CAPILLARY SPHINCTER

cuff of smooth muscle controlling the flow of blood into capillaries; sphincter acts only as on/off valve

PROTEINS

compounds of carbon, hydrogen, oxygen, nitrogen, with small amounts of sulphur, phosphorous, and other elements and found in almost all foodstuffs, but chiefly in beans, lentils, meat, and grains; protein is an essential component of animal diets: in the human diet about 10% of the energy intake must be protein (see AMINO ACIDS)

PROFESSIONAL

a sportsman who plays or competes for pay; creative accounting has enabled many sportsmen to disguise their income and continue competing as amateurs — hence "shamateurs"

PULMONARY CIRCULATION
the blood supply and blood vessels of the lungs

PYRUVIC ACID
the immediate end product of GLYCOLYSIS; when present in excess, is converted into lactic acid in which form it leaves the cell entering the blood

RADIATION
the transfer of heat between two bodies at different temperatures which are not in contact with each other; depends on the 4th power of the temperature gradient and on the absorption/reflection characteristics of the bodies

RIGOR MORTIS
release of membrane calcium into muscle after death activates the contraction machinery, but since ATP is no longer being made, once formed the crossbridges cannot be broken, causing muscle rigidity

S-A NODE
sino-atrial node (see PACEMAKER)

SARCOMERE
the smallest functional subdivision of the contraction machinery

SARCOPLASMIC RETICULUM
network of membranes within the muscle cell one of whose functions is to store calcium, and to release it when stimulated by an action potential; cardiac muscle has a small sarcoplasmic reticulum, smooth muscle has none

SEMI-PERMEABLE MEMBRANE
membrane impermeable to certain substances, but allowing others to pass; cell membranes are all semi-permeable

SKELETAL (OR STRIATED) MUSCLE
type of muscle always attached to bones for the purpose of moving the skeleton; (see also CARDIAC and SMOOTH MUSCLE)

SLOW TWITCH MUSCLE
small muscle fibres specialised for aerobic, endurance activity

SMOOTH MUSCLE
type of muscle found in blood vessels, gastro-intestinal tract, and certain other tissues; generally produces and/or controls flow; never attached to bones or tendons (see also CARDIAC and SKELETAL MUSCLE)

SODIUM
the major positive ION found in the extracellular fluid

SPHINCTER
ring of muscle in small arteries and in the intestine which can close the

tube and stop flow
STROKE VOLUME
the amount of blood pumped by a single contraction of the ventricle;
the volume is adjustable and larger in exercise than at rest
SWEAT
the fluid secreted by the skin for the purposes of evaporative cooling; a
watery protein-free solution containing mainly sodium and chloride
(salt) usually at somewhat lower concentration than in the plasma, but
under appropriate conditions sweat may become virtually salt-free
SYSTEMIC CIRCULATION
the blood vessels serving the whole body, except the lungs
SYSTOLE
the period of the cardiac cycle during which ventricular contraction
(muscle shortening) occurs
SYSTOLIC PRESSURE
the blood pressure during systole, when the ventricles are contracting;
the highest pressure during the cardiac cycle; normally 120 mmHg
TESTOSTERONE
the male sex hormone; an ANABOLIC steroid hormone which
promotes the synthesis of muscle protein; testosterone and synthetic
versions of the hormone are used by sportsmen to build muscle strength
THERMOREGULATION
the processes (both active and passive) by which body temperature is
regulated
TRAINING
the process of repeating a physically demanding task at sufficient
intensity, and often enough to improve performance
VALVES
connective tissue flaps ensuring unidirectional flow of blood; there are
four in the heart and they occur in most veins
VASCULAR RESISTANCE
resistance to flow of the whole vascular system; over 50% is due to the
ARTERIOLES
VEIN
elastic, muscular low pressure blood vessel
VENA CAVA
large vein which empties into the right side of the heart
VENOUS RETURN
amount of blood returning to the heart each minute; equal to the
CARDIAC OUTPUT
VENTRICLE
heavily muscled, high pressure pumping chambers of the heart; there

are two, one left and one right; the former is more muscular than the latter

VENULE
small, elastic low pressure blood vessel

VISCOSITY
measure of a fluid's resistance to flow; viscous fluid is thick and reluctant to flow — like treacle

VO_{2MAX}
the maximum rate at which oxygen can be consumed; affected relatively little by training — appears to be largely genetically determined (see OBLA)

WARM-BLOODED
generally refers to animals whose metabolism produces enough heat to maintain normal body temperature without their depending on heat gained from the environment

WASTES (metabolic)
metabolic wastes include carbon dioxide, lactic acid, adenosine, potassium, heat, etc.; these substances all dilate blood vessels, tending to increase blood flow and wash out the wastes (see LOCAL CONTROL)

WORK
work (w) is performed whenever a force (f) acts over a distance (d): $w = f \times d$; work is expressed in units of Joules or kiloJoules (see JOULE and POWER)

WATT
a measure of power, or the rate of doing work; one Watt = one Joule per second (see JOULE, POWER, WORK)

Index